50-*ish* Reasons

Why actively and purposely
withholding the B.N.B.B.s,
from your body, is a ***really bad idea***.

Sensible-supplementation
of Daily Dietary Habits.

by

Sovereign M. Valentine

https://sovereign-valentine.mykajabi.com/

50-*ish* Reasons

Why actively and purposely withholding the B.N.B.B.s, from your body, is a *really bad idea*.

Sensible-supplementation of Daily Dietary Habits.

by

Sovereign M. Valentine

Author of

Reasons or Results! Performance Nutrition Training
Weighting to Wait
If I Were Her Trainer
Be Your Own Personal Trainer
and
Reasons or Results! Life-long Fat-loss Program & Journal

About The Author

Sovereign Valentine has invested the last decades studying, experimenting and applying science-based, general fitness principles as well as perfecting the nutrition principles contained herein.

After witnessing first-hand, the affects of poor lifestyle choices, within his family and breaking free of the junk food and sugar addiction behaviors himself, he has been refining and practicing what he preaches for more than three-decades. During that time, Sov personally invested tens-of-thousands-of-dollars experimenting to find out what products and ideas are hoaxes and which ones are actually effective and work, with those whom commit to applying them.

Through an intensive and extensive trial-and-error process and by consistently doing what was purported to work he found what really *does* work. He then goes about documenting the results with each client.

In Sov's words, *"There is no longer a mystery to applying nutrition for improved health. The science and art have been figured out...there aren't exceptions...it simply comes down to doing the correct things at the correct times and refining as you go. If you think you're an exception, you're not...that just means you're missing out!"*

Sovereign began his formal training as a health care professional, with a sincere desire to work with athletes. From a combination of formal training and experimenting, he developed a system that *absolutely works*.

Sovereign says, *"If you're putting S.A.D.CR.A.P. in your body and actively, purposely withholding solid nutrition-density, from your body, don't be surprised when your body starts hurting, knagging and breaking down for no apparent reason. IF, on the other hand, you simply want to be shown what to do to feel better than you ever have before, I can help you with that!"*

In 1992 he became a Licensed Massage Therapist, in Washington State. In 1994 he began doing small, informal nutrition presentations, so that others could experience the profound impact that real nutrition has on the body. In 1996 he became a foot and hand reflexologist, as well as an energetic healing master. In 1997 he became a certified hypno-therapist. In 1998 he began training others in hypnotherapy and in 1999 he became the first and only person ever, at The Gabriel Institute, to be certified as a Master Clinical Hypnotherapist. He went on to become certified in Fitness Training, Fitness Therapy, Sports Conditioning, Endurance Conditioning, a Specialist in Performance Nutrition, as well as a Youth Conditioning Specialist, Golf Fitness Instructor, Senior Fitness Specialist, Community Emergency Response Team Member and Emergency First Responder.

Sovereign's thorough understanding of the systems of the body and how they relate to one another is reflected in his ability to fine-tune his client's training and nutritional regimes, for extra-ordinary *Results!* His published works include *Reasons or Results Performance Nutrition Training, Weighting To Wait, Be Your Own Personal Trainer, If I Were Her Trainer,* and *Results! Life-long Fat-loss.*

Foreword

The fitness, nutrition, weight-loss and health improvement industries have been evolving over the last hundred-years, but especially so in the last forty-years, as being overweight and obese, as well as diabetes and all the other *dis*-eases that accompany being overweight have increased to epidemic proportions. While the 'secrets' of improved health and preventive health have evolved, so has the science of how to persuade and convince people to forego their long-term health goals for the immediate payoff of tasty, stimulating junk food (S.A.D.C.R.A.P), which robs the potential for health that improves with time, but likely decreases health on a day-in, day-out basis.

Generally speaking, the amount of health and fitness information is simply crazy. But accurate, science-based information which produces healthy, consistent results that can be maintained over the long haul is simple in nature, but challenging to isolate and replicate. Much of what's out there is simply about spewing marketing and advertising solutions for some problem symptoms (being overweight and in pain) and then saying, *"Here, take this and all your problems will be solved."*

"The truth of the matter, after applying this kind of information for more than three-decades, on both myself and with my clients, is that there truly are good nutritional products that make health, fitness and weight-loss easier, faster and with less effort, but they are few-and-far-between and the general public simply can't tell good products from ineffective ones. That's a part of what I do...assure quality and success through health improvement to prevent and reduce suffering".

In the United States right now, the right people are doing the right research to help you get real *Results!* At the same time, most food products and dietary-supplements for sale really have little nutrition at all, resulting in a lot of missed opportunities by people whom could have gotten better *Results!* but to this day don't know why they don't know.

When you hear the words 'fad diet', what they're talking about is either a good program that people picked away at, until there wasn't any relevant nutritional content left (requires lifestyle change). Or, the program promised weight-loss, fitness and athletic results without exercise and nutritional-density, to begin with. With any health and fitness program, if the amount of nutritional-density isn't increased and isn't provided to your body consistently, you simply won't stick with it since there's no pay off to your chemistry of the brain and body, without additional, consistent nutrition-density. True nutrition-density works so well, when put in the body, that it overrides and benefits a person thinks they get from consuming S.A.D.C.R.A.P./junk food.

Secondly, any program that suggests you can improve your health in all ways without adding nutrition-density is a pipe dream. The body is made of nutrition and as nutrition-density is decreased, regardless of the period of time it occurs and so will the level of health decrease proportionately. Some kind of resistance-training [and] cardiovascular/aerobic-exercise should be included in and health-building program (start where you can) but nutrition-density, (what I coined as the B.N.B.B.s), makes up 80% of the results you get or miss out on...do all the exercise and training you want, without the B.N.B.B.s you're not coming close to your potential and the more you exercise the more injuries you'll likely experience (seemingly out of nowhere/mysteriously), as a result of not maintaining your body.

A true secret is finding a nutrition coach whom has your overall health in mind (not just short-term results) [your health should be improving and you should be feeling better as time goes on] and a nutrition coach whom has enough expertise to not only design an amazingly effective program, but one whom knows how to adjust the program to you for most effectiveness. Many nutrition trainers can design a program, but many don't know how to adjust the program if progress slows down or progress hits a plateau (accountability for both the client and the trainer). *This is the second part of what I do.*

One of the things that makes me so effective as a nutrition coach is that I've been doing this so long, that when a client isn't getting results, I can narrow it down to whether it has something to do with the 1) Whole-foods, 2) Functional-foods or 3) B.N.B.B.s.

There simply aren't any mysteries to healthy, sustainable health to me anymore. A majority of trainers don't stick with the industry long enough to find out what *they didn't know*...I have.

I think this book provides enough evidence that most people aren't getting enough nutrition-density, from the food (they are consuming), as well as lays out a clear plan of action that you can start applying this week.

When you apply these tactics, in the way I show you here, you and those whom know you will be blown away by the *Results!* you are getting. This book is for people whom want the results that speak for themselves...anyone can get some results in the short-run...every 'die-it' will produce some kind of results in the short-run, but most quick, fitness programs erode the physical health after leaving you malnourished, tired, exhausted and depleted...*resulting in decreased health and vitality.*

Any health-building fitness program should leave you feeling lighter, clearer, relaxed, rejuvenated and more vital than when you started, as well as free of all cravings and any attraction to junk food.

Apply this information and you will be so glad you did...*I promise.*

Read this book now; start getting better today and I look forward to seeing and hearing how good you feel about the *Results!* you are getting!

Once you've read the material, if you're the type to recognize what is real and not just the next fad and if you're willing to commit and follow through until the end, *I'll be there with you every step of the way.*

Acknowledgments

I have not attempted to cite, in the text, all the authorities and sources in the preparation of this book. To do so would require more space than is practical, in order to effectively serve you whom apply this information. The list would include departments of the federal government, libraries, industrial institutions, web sources and many individuals, as well as my personal-experiences and those of my clients, since the late 1980's.

Inspiration was contributed by all those before me whom succeeded as best they could with the information they had at the time, as well as all those after me whom will improve upon this information to make the lives of others better. This book is a culmination of hundreds-of-books I've read, thousands-of-hours of experimentation and thousands-of-hours of observing the why, how and where of my own and others' successes and failures.

A Word From The Author

Do it!

This is a *do it* book…read it, learn it…*do it.* If you don't apply it as instructed, you'll miss out. Reading this book provides the information, but is not the same as doing. E-mail me and let me know you want to be shown how to get started and I'll help you every step of the way.

I work to make a living, but I live to see you get *Results!*

Sovereign Michael Valentine,

Montana, December 2019

Disclaimer

This book is designed to provide information about the subject matter covered. It is produced and sold with the understanding that the publisher and author are not engaged in rendering neither medical diagnosis nor treatment. If you need medical help, go get it. It is not the purpose of this manual to reprint all the information that is otherwise available from other health professionals but to complement, amplify and supplement other texts. *50-ish Reasons* is neither a cure-all nor a quick-fix for poor lifestyle habits or tendencies. Anyone whom commits to personal accountability for their health must expect to re-direct some time, energy and money without any guarantee for specific benefits within a fixed time frame. *Nature works at her own pace.*

Every effort has been made to make this book as complete and accurate as possible. However, there may be mistakes both typographical and in content. Therefore, this book should be used as a general guide and not as the ultimate source of health and nutritional information. Your uniqueness will shine through as you succeed.

The purpose of this book is to educate and inform. The very best results will come from participation. Neither the publisher nor the author shall have responsibility to any person or entity with respect to any loss or damage caused by or alleged to be caused directly or indirectly by the information contained in this book.

This book is not meant to replace the advice or treatments prescribed by your doctor, but rather to accompany your physician's advice. It is not meant to encourage medical treatment of illness or disease or any medical problem by the layperson. It is meant to inform you and open you to health choices that are available to those whom seek a broader knowledge. Any application of the ideas set forth in this book is at the applicant's discretion and sole risk. If you are under a doctor's care for any condition, she or he can advise you *about information she or he is familiar with and which she or he has personally experienced.*

The information in this book is neither diagnostic nor prescriptive. It is informational only. The data and information contained herein are based upon information from various peer-reviewed, published and unpublished sources and merely represent training, experience, health and nutrition literature and practices summarized.

Neither the publisher nor the author of this book makes any warranties, expressed or implied regarding the currency, completeness or scientific accuracy or validity of this information nor does it warrant the fitness of the information for any particular purpose. It is intended to provide helpful and informative material on the subjects addressed in the publication. It is sold with the understanding that the publisher and author are not engaged in rendering medical, health, or any other kind of personal professional services in this book. The publisher and author specifically disclaim all responsibility for any liability, loss or risk, personal or otherwise which is incurred as a consequence, directly or indirectly, from the use and application of any of the contents of this book.

For Medical Providers:

One of the single greatest suggestions I can make regarding consideration of research on dietary-supplements being done and published, nowadays…whether in favor of or against supplementing, *dig a little deeper*…often I have found that published research e.g. *"Vitamin A toxicity for pregnant women,"* or *"Beta Carotene increases smoker's mortality,"* or *"Chromium promotes fat-loss,"* or *"Vitamin E increases mortality rate,"* and topics of that nature, often do not fully disclose in a forthcoming manner, whether the researchers used synthetic, extracted or concentrated food-form supplements…*a 'detail' that can make all the difference in the dietary-supplements being a success and whether the results were measurable and noticeable in blood chemistry lab results.*

So, it's important, when reading those kinds of studies to discern whether the kind of nutrients used were man-made or concentrated food-form…otherwise, the conclusions and assumptions, especially in this regard is only relevant to the type of supplement given to the human subjects whom participated in the studies.

In my research, and contrasted with my personal-experiences, the results reported in supposed peer-reviewed articles often promote themselves at the holy-grail of scientific information available to the medical and scientific profession, while simultaneously failing to be forthright about the standard quality of the nutritional supplements used in the studies…e.g. just because it's called 'Beta carotene' or 'Chromium' in a study or abstract doesn't mean that what was used in such studies even came close to what nature intends when using those words…yes, I'm saying the researchers use substances 'call them' by names known as nutrients all knowing that the real definitions of those names didn't come close to being included in such studies, yet purport the results to the professional and consumer market as if the real ingredients were used simply because the words were used.

What a shame.

The order or priority of the nutrients used by each person's body may have variation, (one person's body may use more of a particular nutrient(s) than another) and each person's body prioritizes particular nutrients differently (e.g. one person might use Zinc before Iron or vice-versa), but everyone's body [requires] and is made of the same basic nutritional building blocks (B.N.B.B.s).

In practical terms, this means ***put nutrition in your body and let nature take over.*** Not all supplements are created equal nor safe to consume. To learn what kind my decades of experience have steered me toward, contact me at the email in the appendix for your complimentary consultation. You'll be glad you did.

Eye-opener

In 2017, an article was published entitled *Health effects of dietary risks in 195 countries, 1990-2017, a systematic analysis for the Global Burden of Disease Study 2017.* The study is a collaboration between 125 professionals and more than 100 consultants, schools of medicine and health organizations.

What the study found:

In 2017, 11-million deaths and 255-million DALYs (*Disability-adjusted life year,* a measurement of overall *dis*-ease burden, expressed as the number of years lost due to poor health, disability or early death), were attributable to inadequate nutrition-intake…in other words, no country is getting enough nutrition-density (B.N.B.B.s), even when they have the income to do so.

The most common missing Whole-foods that could provide some nutrition-density are fruits, vegetables, grains, nuts, seeds and fish containing good-fats. The study defined the optimal level of intake as the level of risk exposure that **minimizes the risk from** ***all causes of death.***

Consumption of nearly all healthy foods and nutrients was not enough. In conjunction with not putting enough nutrition-density in the body, too little healthy food consumption (daily intake of S.A.D.C.R.A.P.), exceeds the optimal level…*a double-whammy.*

Observations worldwide show that the effects for most of the dietary interventions to get people to put more nutrition-density in their body, are far below the level required to achieve optimal health.

In other words, regardless of the interventions to improve the diet of all populations of all 195 countries (in order to lower the incidence of chronic and non-communicable *dis*-eases), none of them have improved the amount of nutrition-density to optimize health in any country. So…where are the people who are getting enough nutrition-density from their diet???

Table of Contents

Table of Contents continued

Definitions

1) Whole-foods: Fresh food with the least amount of processing, packaging, preservation, (other than fermented-foods), chemicals, salt, sugar, fake fats, etc. *Food.*

2) Functional-foods; Foods designed to elicit a certain physiological response at certain times: *e.g. stabilize blood sugar level, recovery post-workout, replace electrolytes.* Generally speaking, functional–foods are foods which have a higher [consistency] level of nutrition, than non Functional-foods and work faster to deliver a consistent amount of nutrition-density, that makes all the difference in the world, during time-sensitive events and activities, such as fat-loss and sports events.

3) B.N.B.B.s: Basic Nutritional Building Blocks; concentrated food in tablet, capsule and powder form, including:

The B.N.B.B.s include ultra high-quality:

- Protein powder,

- Multi-vitamin/mineral,

- Vitamin B-Complex,

- Vitamin C-Complex

- Vitamin E-Complex

- Good Fats

- *Pro*-biotics

- Dietary Fiber

- Clean drinking water

4) *De-generation: The slow, [often with seemingly sudden onset] process of gradual and preventable breakdown, of the essential systems and capabilities of the body.

*When the body doesn't have adequate B.N.B.B.s consistently consumed/delivered and it begins to break down, malfunction, dys-function, manifest syndromes, symptoms, signs, aches, pains, and includes fat-gain.

5) *Dis-ease: The symptoms, mal-functions, dys-functions, syndromes, aches, pains and signs letting us know the process of de-generation is well on its way because the cells need the B.N.B.B.s...dis-ease(s), are considered "normal" and "average", in much of the medical community, to those professionals whom don't know about the B.N.B.B.s [through first-hand, personal-experience]. Meaning, unless they are putting them in their own body, they really don't have first-hand experience with them.

*Italics added to [de-generative] and [dis-ease] as a reminder that they are 'processes' which can be interrupted, rather than 'things we have to live with or have no influence over.

6) S.A.D.C.R.A.P.=Standard American Diet of Continuously & Repetitively Advertised Products:

S.A.D.C.R.A.P. includes, but is not limited to:

• Soda pop

• Carbonated beverage

• Candy

• Chips

• Ice cream

• Caffeine

• Alcohol

• Tobacco

Anything with partially-hydrogenated oil, artificial fats, artificial sweetener, artificial coloring, artificial preservatives.

7) Complete Recovery Drink: Must be a combination of protein & carbohydrate in a ratio of 2.7 (divide protein grams by carbohydrate grams), re-fuel the body following exercise, training, competition as well as recover from injury, illness, *de*-generation & *dis*-ease.

8) The *"Black-forest of chasing symptoms"*: Refers to the process whereby people taking note of or being diagnosed with a particular health problem, symptom, sign, syndrome and/or *de*-generative *dis*-ease and so forth, cover up the underlying symptoms with medication,..only to have another symptom appear from the medication itself, which in-turn gets covered up with another medication…which, in-turn gets covered up by another medication…eventually, to find their health so *de*-generated and mixed-up that things seem bleak and hopeless.

9) Search-and-Consume Mode: When someone has waited too long to eat or drink and they reach for whatever will get them some energy the fastest…often S.A.D.C.R.A.P…which often leads to a sharp increase in energy followed by a sharp decrease in energy…leading to yet another 'search-and-consume-mode'…which cumulatively and ultimately takes one into the "Black-forest of *de*-generative *dis*-ease".

Every cell of the body requires the B.N.B.B.s to maintain, repair and rejuvenate themselves. There are no exceptions. One can't know if they have enough of them until they do have enough and things that seemed normal simply go away.

Often people attending one of my lectures or reading one of my books will ask, *"Yay, but what about my…?"* What's the answer?

The B.N.B.B.s!

Yes, some of the cells and systems require other things in addition, but you want to make sure the basics are in place instead of skipping the basics and substituting other things which I refer to as accessories.

Just like breathing air.

Just like drinking water.

Just like eating food.

Every cell requires them.

One might wonder… *"I have such and such,"* or *"I was diagnosed with this or that…what should I take?"*

Begin with the B.N.B.B.s.

Build upon the B.N.B.B.s.

Every cell requires them.

A few words on weight-loss/fat-loss…

"Until we boldly separate the two concepts of food & nutrition from one another, there will always be confusion, debate and resulting subpar nutrition in the body, resulting in subpar body composition (too much fat). The confusion lies in the 'one or the other' debate (food or dietary-supplements?). Food doesn't necessarily provide consistent enough nutrition and nutrition-density isn't necessarily provided by what we call/think of as food."
-Sov

For those of us in the nutrition industry, with enough field experience to reflect upon (from the inside out), the relative strengths and weaknesses of the nutrition models, we go through and the information provided to us as health professionals for our certification(s), we realize there is a vast ethical, moral and cognitive dissonance between:

What the consumer of nutrition marketing information wants to believe is intuitive, in terms of what they need to do to lose 'weight' and build health (what we think is right action):

e.g. "Eat less to lose weight."

What the consumer of weight-loss marketing information wants to believe is intuitive in terms of what they need to do to burn 'fat' (what we think is right action):

e.g. "As long as I weigh less and get smaller I don't care how it happens."

How much of what is marketed to the consumer of weight-loss marketing information to personal-trainers, fitness trainers and the like pick up and believe to be credible, safe and effective in the long-run (for their clients), and in turn apply or get their clients to 'do' as ways of attempting to ratify their own value of service, (promise certain results to gain a client followed with no way of holding themselves accountable to potential weight-loss goals let alone health improvements for the clients):

e.g. "As long as the client loses weight and gets smaller they won't know if they have done it safely or not and the trainers don't care as long as they get paid."

What is quick, convenient, mediocre in terms of safety, noticeable and yet un-sustainable by the lay-person vs what is sustainably fast, safe, easy, noticeable as well as clinically measurable as health promoting in the short and long-run for improvement of body composition as well as long-term health:

e.g. The main focus is on the client losing weight in the first six-weeks, regardless whether it is safe and healthy or not."

And finally, the fitness professional's ability to discern between what is weight-loss marketing 'hype' (advertising disguised as information or science to keep a consumer wanting to lose weight as long as possible…keep them buying stuff which promises weight-loss, delivers little and makes the body crave things which cause weight gain):

e.g. Even many personal trainers don't know if the information and direction they are providing is safe for their clients but they don't know how to measure 'safe' let alone hold themselves accountable to ethical practices."

[And its application should therefore be avoided both by consumers and by fitness professionals due to short-term weight-loss in trade for long-term health distortion]:

e.g. Just because someone loses weight doesn't mean they got healthier in the process…health should be the first priority followed by fat-loss…neither are exclusive...and what is practical, applicable, re-producible science (and its application should not only be adhered to by consumers and health professionals due to short and long-term, sustainable fat-loss, but also for clinically measurable and documentable improvements in bio-chemical markers, *e.g. blood pressure, total cholesterol, HDL, LDL, triglyceride levels, blood sugar, insulin sensitivity, etc.* for the top ten *de*-generative *dis*-eases of our time, e.g. heart *dis*-ease, diabetes, stroke, obesity, etc.):

e.g. When one burns fat safely the chemistry of the body improves and the overall health improves and can be measured by your physician...if the above markers didn't improve there may be too much emphasis placed on 'weight-loss' first, without regard for health, which is the metabolically and physiologically sound way to burn fat and yet, largely neither marketed nor promoted nor understood, by much of the average fitness professional and even less understood by the weight-loss consumer market?

e.g. Based on my experiences working elbow-to-elbow with other trainers, "I believe relatively few fitness professionals know the difference between weight-loss and fat-loss or the differences in facilitating the two,"...for example, a few of the many common and misunderstood concepts regarding weight-loss:

• Low fat diets,

• Good vs. bad fats,

• Calorie restriction,

• High protein diets,

• Low carbohydrate diets,

• Attempts at 'starving the fat'

• Frequency of meals and snacks,

• Withholding of nutrition-density,

• Quality vs. quantity of fat consumption,

• Exercise without application of nutrition,

• Attempts at weight-loss without application of nutrition and

• Attempts at weight-loss success through deprivation and the like.

e.g. The things which don't work in the long-run.

The above list has been shown to produce short-term weight-loss (loss of lean mass along with some body fat), and accompanying disintegration of critical blood-chemistry markers of health *e.g. blood pressure, total cholesterol, HDL, LDL, triglyceride levels, blood sugar, insulin sensitivity, etc.* followed by re-bound affects (re-gaining the weight and more):

e.g. The diet-market promotes the concept of the quick-fix without regard for the long-term affects...taking advantage of people's desperation while the practical, applicable, re-producible science:

● Decreases body fat,

● Improves lean mass,

● Improves bone mass and

● Improves blood pressure, total cholesterol, HDL, LDL, triglyceride levels, blood sugar, insulin sensitivity, etc.

e.g. Do it correctly and your whole life will improve and get better with time.

The themes repeated throughout this book

are done so purposely and with great intent,

for the people whom need them most,

and are by no stretch of the imagination a coincidence.

Insight

It's not uncommon that when the average person seeks professional-coaching, they are afraid of what they'll be told (*"Don't take away my ice cream..."*). They're afraid to be told anything different than what they want to believe or want to believe is true or what is convenient in support of their established-habits (which are merely actions that have been chosen, repeated and driven/charged by emotions, which have also been chosen to be utilized). They're afraid that they'll be told to do things that interfere with the lifestyle they have created which got them to a place the no longer want to be at or that they are no longer satisfied with. *People like to hear (their) ideas are correct and they are right even when they aren't.* There's a vast difference between being fit, healthy and vital and being right. People are so "right" today that 80% of the population is overweight...how can we be fat and out of shape and wrong?

In this way, the greatest challenge for trainers and coaches is helping people understand, comprehend and correlate how their thinking has gotten them to a place they want to get away from.

The very best coaches introduce ideas in such a way that a person can feel "right" learning, never noticing that what they are learning might be the opposite of what/how they wish things were or how they insist things are even as they get further and further from the best versions of themselves.

You'll likely get some new ideas, herein...maybe they sound like old ideas...but, the difference is in applying them to yourself versus debating, theorizing, hypothesizing, processing yet, never applying. Getting super-fit and healthy is easy when you just do what works and don't interfere in your own process.

Some points are stated repeatedly throughout this book in every conceivable manner, in response to every question I've heard since I started experimenting with nutrition, since age 12...to leave absolutely no question, no matter which angle you perceive the points, what I mean by what I'm saying...*unequivocal clarity.*

These are not just ideas...these are proven principles I've been applying with myself for close to thirty-five years and with my family, friends and clients for twenty-five plus years.

The only thing that can get in your way now is what you tell yourself about this information.

Go for it!

Clarity

Consumers and professionals alike often still think the idea of dietary-supplements is *debatable*. Anyone who *lacks personal-experience,* with successful supplementation, can certainly be in that corner. But, that's the way everything is…*those who lack success and experience attempt to talk others out of having success…or believe that their ideas and opinions are the same as facts.* Every industry is this way, regardless of a person's professional status and education.

Steven R. Gundry, MD, author of *The Plant Paradox*, puts it this way:

"Let me tell you why nutrient supplementation is a critical-component…I can choose no better source to convince you of that than the United States Federal Government. Here is the actual wording in U.S. Senate Document 74-264: **The alarming fact is that foods-fruits, vegetables and grains – now being raised on millions of acres of land that no longer contains enough of certain needed nutrients, are starving us-no matter how much we eat of them** (in other words, full but empty…fed but not fueled…even fat, but under-nourished).

Dr. Gundry goes on to ask lecture attendees what year they think this was written?

Any guess, when the soil was recognized as nutritionally-depleted?

Answer: 1936!

Chapter One

Most people have multiple reasons overlapping...

Want to *feel better?* For the most part we are literally taught, by the media, to eat what we are convinced to think makes us *feel* 'good' in the moment (e.g. excess sugar, excess salt, rancid fried-fats, ice cream, caffeine, alcohol and other chemicals useless to human physiological health) versus what we know is healthier for us, then ignore the effects they are having on the body from moment-to-moment. And yes, when the body begins to *de*-generate, fail, breakdown and hurt we can get medicine to cover up the symptoms, so we won't notice that we are aging and dying prematurely, because those problems we are having are *"...within normal limits,"* (and part of the normal aging process, for malnourished people)...for Americans whom eat junk and fast-energy food and beverage (S.A.D.C.R.A.P.)., *while withholding the B.N.B.B.s and substituting Whole-foods with S.A.D.C.C.R.A.P.!*

The following are some reasons why you might choose to supplement your Whole-foods, with the B.N.B.B.s. To review from the introduction, here's what I mean by the B.N.B.B.s. Notice there are seven:

The B.N.B.B.s include ultra high quality:

1. Protein,

2. Multi-vitamin/mineral,

3. Vitamin B-Complex,

4. Vitamin C-Complex

5. Vitamin E-Complex

6. Good-fats and

7. *Pro*-biotics

Notice there are 7 different B.N.B.B.s. How you decide which ones to take is to start with the top two (protein and multi-vitamin/mineral). If that is the extent of your spending budget, start there and do it consistently each month. That's where I started. If you don't have the same constraints and you want to maximize the benefits, work your way through the list. The third one is B-Complex, the fourth is C, the fifth is E and so on, finishing with good-fats and *pro*-biotics. You get and take as many as you can afford to do consistently...*consistency is more important than taking all 7 some of the time.* Take 2 or 3 or 4 or all 7…it's up to you, but however many you take, take them consistently, so budget accordingly, so you can accurately measure the results you get. Don't change the priority/order! Start at the top and add on the way down the list.

The order the body uses the B.N.B.B.s is prioritized by nature, not me.

Over the decades of doing this work, both personally and professionally, this is the order I have noticed works best, based on how [nature and the body] prioritizes nutrient use and which ones are needed more than others. In other words, don't change the order. As your budget allows, do them in that order and do whatever you can do (consistently). Consistency of two-or-more is more important than hit-and-miss of the 7 key B.N.B.B.s.

On March 15, 2017 Dr. Oz said, *"Just one supplement has so many benefits."*

What I consider a complete nutrition program and what I measure progress by is three-part: 1) Whole-foods 2) Functional-foods and 3) The B.N.B.B.s.

Each is defined in the definitions area in the front of this book. If someone isn't getting the *Results* they say they want, I look at how much, if any, of these three they are doing well. If none, or one or two of them are in place, there's room for improvement and that's part of what I've been helping people do the last couple-decades.

Reason 1. Want to *prevent unnecessary aging?*

When the body doesn't get enough B.N.B.B.s, on a day-in and day-out basis, the body heads toward wearing itself out, faster (at the cellular level) than it is able to repair, rebuild, regenerate and maintain itself. The net result is that people whom get the B.N.B.B.s every day, consistently end up getting more compliments that they look younger than they are and they feel younger than other people their age.

Reason 2. Want to *look 10-15 years younger?*

People whom don't get the B.N.B.B.s everyday may not be even getting enough nutrition to keep the body healthy, let alone to affect how they look. The appearance of the hair, skin, nails and even the bone structure of the face are directly affected by the level of B.N.B.B.s you get and how frequently you put them in your body (how consistent you are). Put them in everyday and you'll always look younger than you are as well as younger than the average person of your biological age. And yes, you will continue to have a younger, more youthful appearance. The longer you take them the effects are cumulative. *Start now, be consistent.*

Reason 3. Want to *increase your spendable income?*

I've told people for years the stories of clients whom come back to me after applying these B.N.B.B. tactics on a regular basis. The net result is that they say things like, *"You won't believe what happened..."*

Not only do they have the fat-burning, health-building benefits I go on and on about, but one way or another they 'mysteriously' find an improved lifestyle, within a short period of time, for no apparent recognizable or seemingly associated reasons.

In the decades of experience applying and experimenting with this stuff, I have found that people whom don't apply the B.N.B.B.s seem to be under-functioning, at a brain-capacity level...meaning the front of the brain, the part responsible for higher functioning, recognition of opportunity and planning/goal programming requires higher amounts of nutrition-density (B.N.B.B.s), than does making emotional decisions, which may feel good in the moment, but lack long-term pay off or goal achievement.

As people apply these strategies, their upper-brain (pre-frontal cortext functioning), seems to 'come back online' resulting in greater cognitive, emotional and creative capacity, as well as greater capacity to recognize opportunity that often has been right in front of their nose all along.

Reason 4. Earn more money:

Ohio State University research has found that people whom reduced their Body Mass Index Score (BMI), by 10 points, saw their net worth rise by $12,000. –September 2005 *Money Magazine.*

Did you know there was a study at Cleveland State University that showed that people whom exercise, at least three times per week, earn 10% more than those whom don't? In the 30 or so years of doing my personal training business, I've seen this over and over. Often, people whom have never exercised consistently begin to notice their career and lifestyle improving in relation to the consistency with which they apply nutrition and exercise. Out of seemingly nowhere, the more consistent they are with their habits, the more opportunities appear for them. So, in order to afford yourself the B.N.B.B.s, first you must afford them!

How much would 10% more income allow you to invest in your own health and fitness? If you earned 10% more, wouldn't that pay for the three parts of your nutrition and then some?

Reason 5. Want to have a *better, more properly responsive immune system?*

People whom don't take the B.N.B.B.s, on a daily basis, often exhibit an under-functioning or over-functioning immune system...*something is off.* In other words, people may get cold, flu and infections throughout the year and consider that 'normal'. Others may have an over-functioning immune system in that they develop allergies, reactions, skin sensitivities and auto-immune type problems.

In both cases, symptoms subside as the chemistry of the immune system begins getting what it needs to build itself up, from the inside out. The immune system is literally made up of and from the B.N.B.B.s.

Opportunistic *dis*-eases are bugs that make themselves at home in bodies which don't have adequate immune defense; things like staph, colds, flu, viruses. People whom don't have enough B.N.B.B.s on board are more vulnerable to opportunistic bugs.

Acquired-immunity is when the immune system is able to notice, recognize and respond to invaders quickly and effectively, without delay. A person whom doesn't have enough B.N.B.B.s will not likely have as strong acquired immunity and responsive immunity as one whom does.

Think of the immune system as a group of soldiers. Do you want your soldiers to be tired and hungry or rested and well fed, prepared for anything?

Dr. Bruce Miller D.D.S., C.N.S. says, *"Turn your immune system up as high as you can get it due to a phenomenal increase in antibiotic resistant bacteria."*

Back in 1996 The World Health Organization said, *"The World is on the brink of global crisis with infectious disease. As more and more bacteria become antibiotic resistant, your only hope is going to be a powerful, strong immune system."*

Although anti-biotics cost so much to produce that less are being developed and made by pharmaceutical companies, while more bugs are becoming anti-biotic resistant. Another option is to build up your own resistance to opportunistic bugs, in the environment. Even if a person does get sick, studies have shown that people whom have a surplus of nutrition-density, in their body get well faster, stay in the hospital for a shorter length of time and have lower medical bills...*this has been studied and documented many times.*

Reason 6: Want to *increase your athletic performance by 20%-50%?*

Athletic ability and capability are the result of cumulative good health, which all begins at the cellular level...*which is a make-it-or-break-it proposition, depending whether you put the B.N.B.B.s in your body or choose to consciously skip them.* I tell people they can get a 20% improvement, in sports performance and truthfully that's a conservative claim. Time-and-time-again, I see the speed and effectiveness of improvement, by simply making a few minor adjustments in one's nutritional-regime. *By simply adding high quality B.N.B.B.s to their regime.* Remember the three-parts of a complete nutrition program? 1) Whole-foods 2) Functional-foods and 3) B.N.B.B.s.

Whether a beginning child or professionally competitive, adult athlete or anywhere in between, most people think that nutrition won't make much of a difference. (*Hint, hint...that means they haven't applied it correctly, before).* It's a crime that what most athletes consider "ability" is a relative-term...*relative to the quality of nutrition they are habitually putting in their body day-in and day-out.*

What I consider a complete nutrition program and what I measure progress by is three-part: 1) Whole-foods 2) Functional-foods and 3) B.N.B.B.s. Each is defined in the introduction of this book. If someone isn't getting the results, they say they want, I look at how much, if any, of these three they are doing correctly or skipping.

Often, folks think they have passed their prime or they just weren't gifted...*until they get the B.N.B.B.s their body has been unwittingly asking for all along.*

In the Winter/Spring 2017 issue of *Boulder* (Colorado) magazine an article entitled, *Gaining the Performance Edge,* San Millan describes similar sports nutrition tactics and says, "*What we can do for the recreational athlete is improve performance by 50%."*

Side note: All the dietary-supplements, Functional-foods, sports supplements and B.N.B.B.s, which I suggest in my private practice, are completely pure and clean, free of any impurities that could disqualify a competitive athlete or professional, as well as all the way to the International Olympic Level. Most dietary-supplement companies cannot claim this and a lot of athletes have been disqualified for impure, low quality supplements, after having trained enough to compete at the international level.

Reason 7. Want to *turn your body into a fat-burning machine?*

The body deficient of the B.N.B.B.s will have trouble burning body-fat, no matter how much or how little exercise they are doing...sustaining any fat-loss is unlikely without adequate nutrition-density surplus in the body. The body short on the B.N.B.B.s may not only crave the food which builds fat, but stores fat without the ability to reverse the effects, by burning the fat (insulin-resistance). You can't outrun poor nutrition with exercise, especially when insulin-resistance is a factor, indicated by excess body fat. Eating the B.N.B.B.s on a daily basis liberates body fat for energy as a result of balancing the blood chemistry thereby sensitizing the receptors to insulin.

One client asked, *"How can you be full, but still feel hungry?"*

Answer: Inadequate B.N.B.B.s.

One of the greatest misconceptions I have found people to have over the years is that all they have to do is reduce how much they eat and they'll lose 'weight' and become healthier (calories-in/calories-out).

In reality, if you want to lose weight (burn fat) easier than you ever have before, prevent cravings, promote your health and vitality overall and sustain that weight without gaining it back, I suggest making sure you get enough Whole-foods, Functional-foods and B.N.B.B.s in your body, on a daily basis. *You may describe the results you get as nothing less than remarkable.*

Truth being what it is, I have found over the last two-or-three decades that the single greatest factor in how quickly and easily one burns fat and rebuilds their health, from the inside out, is directly dependent on stabilizing blood sugar levels and how nutritionally-dense one's daily eating habits are, as well as how much good Whole-foods, Functional-foods and B.N.B.B.s they put in their body, on a daily basis.

The people whom think they 'know better' are too smart to take supplements or skip, skimp, substitute or in any other way compromise their own nutritional fat-burning regime are the folks whom work out for months, at a time, losing very little fat and in a lot of cases continue to gain more fat! They say they *"tried"* exercise and it doesn't work...they *"...look at food and it goes to their hips,"*...they're the one exception to exercise and nutrition...they are on a constant search for the mysterious reason they can't burn fat...but, never stick to a program that emphasizes nutrition-density, first and foremost.

You can't outrun poor nutrition with exercise!

While on the other hand, the people whom heed this advice return time and time again saying, *"You won't believe what happened!"* and *"It's happening just like you said it would!"*

It comes down to being coachable, beginning to end versus trying to work out personal issues by doing the opposite of what is suggested!

The amount of food or calories is [not] as important as how much actual nutrition-density (vitamins, minerals, enzymes and unnamed/unknown co-factors), you consume and how stabilized your blood sugar is, on average. When the nutrition is there, people can eat a lot more food and still burn fat-lose weight. The nutritionally-dense food itself aids in the fat-burning process...*it facilitates the liberation of stored fat as energy...***the key being how**

much nutrition-density you consistently put [in your body], whereas the diet low in nutrition-density will get stored as fat and the fat just stays stored…a one-way street…mainly due to lack of stability of blood sugar…sharp swings in blood sugar equates to stored fat that doesn't get burned during exercise of any variety, intensity or duration…*insulin-resistance.*

Calories do not equate to nutrient-density – The International Sports Sciences Association notes a study done at Syracuse University found numerous nutritional deficiencies, among athletes, some of whom were eating as many as 14,000 calories a day; *Jerzy Meduski, MD re: nutritional biochemistry.*

So, even if you are eating what you think is enough calories, you're likely missing key nutrients that affect performance. **Calories do not equal nutrition-density, but reducing calories does reduce the amount of nutrition-density you get! A paradox. A Catch-22.**

So, if they aren't getting enough nutrition-density, with 14,000 calories, how do people think they'll get enough nutrition with less food? (as in dieting). Yes, less activity means even less calories…**think about it.**

Reason 8. Want to *take control of your health once and for all?*

If you're like me, you may have all kinds of the health problems to begin with. You may have been getting 'treated' with medical care all along and may even be on some medications with unexplainable health challenges that never seem to go away. Believe it or not, that's common with people whom haven't had enough nutrition-density, on a consistent enough basis, for their particular needs.

Simply put the B.N.B.B.s in every day, and let nature do the rest!

Simple!

Reason 9. Faster recovery:

Want to *assure the greatest chances of recovery from incidents in life which cannot be planned for?* e.g. *unexpected surgeries, illness, accidents, traumas, etc.* The body that has a surplus of the B.N.B.B.s will recover faster, and be more resistant to infection.

Reason 10. General health assurance:

General health requires that the body have a "surplus" or nutritional savings-account, *if you will,* to repair, maintain and rebuild the body at the cellular level. In the case of accidents, injuries, illness and surgery the body requires even higher amounts, to make up for the increased need by the body...*and it needs it to be in place ahead of time.* Makes sense, right? -If you're going to drive your car harder than usual, you'll need more fuel and engine fluids on board before you need them. If you procrastinate maintenance, the engine may break down from the inside out.

If you want to assure your greatest chances of optimal recovery get Whole-foods, Functional-foods and the B.N.B.B.s in your body every day, so that if anything does happen your body is ready.

In my experience, I was told by numerous medical professionals that it would take five-weeks to recover from a surgery I had. To their surprise, *I was back to work in 10-days!*

Let's think about this for a minute...

I. The body is made of the B.N.B.B.s.

II. If the body doesn't get enough B.N.B.B.s it doesn't have what it needs to...

a) ***Halt the dis-ease or de-generation,*** of the body systems and capabilities,

b) ***Prevent further damage*** from previous inadequate consumption of the B.N.B.B.s,

c) To ***Reverse prior damage*** from inadequate B.N.B.B.s. and

d) ***Repair, rebuild and maintain*** the fundamental systems and capabilities of the body…*the point where personal performance will significantly improve beyond what you thought you were capable of!*

III. Getting enough of the things that make up the very structure of the body (B.N.B.B.s), makes for a healthier version of you.

IV. Healthier version of you means better health *assurance* for you!

Medical 'treatments' are a monopoly of their own...there's a *presupposition* there...that a person has to *de*-generate to a certain degree before 'treatment' is appropriate...meaning we have to wait for the body to 'breakdown' (enough) for the treatment to be applied, while the underlying nutritional-deficiency is still active.

No one is allowed to medically "treat" unless they are licensed for their scope of practice to do so. Sooooo,..what about the people whom aren't totally healthy or satisfied with their health and vitality, but they aren't considered sick enough to be treated? I was in that category. Nutrition isn't a "treatment" since the body itself is made out of nutrition-density...take away every bit of nutrition from the body and there isn't a body at all!...yes, people and organizations are trying to patent each person's cells and DNA the same way they have done with fruits and vegetables, so they can charge the farmer for every piece of produce they sell...a monopoly. Would it make sense to withhold (purposely make absent from the body and brain), nutrition information to the professions whom provide medical treatment to people whom didn't know that their body is made up of nutrition?...until the body breaks down enough that the body MUST be 'treated' medically? *Think about it,* physicians get two-hours of nutrition training, *if* they take the elective class during medical school. The same medical school that are literally funded by the pharmaceutical companies? Isn't that a conflict of interest? Some doctors go outside the primary medical system to get nutrition training...especially if they have had health problems that their own skill set couldn't help.

Reason 11. Digestive problems?

The digestive system is just one of the many systems of the body, which is supposed to work in a cooperative and synergistic fashion, with the other systems of the body.

When the body doesn't have enough B.N.B.B.s the digestive system will suffer, partly because the digestive system *itself* requires adequate nutritional building blocks to maintain *itself*...the system responsible for distributing the B.N.B.B.s!

I was a person whom had digestive problems, from early in life. Pretty much every problem from the top to the bottom.

If you're taking any kind of medication for your digestive system and would prefer to address the underlying problem rather than chasing symptoms around the Black-forest, *ask me for help*. I don't know if it'll work as good for you as it did for me, but what do you have to lose? *No risk.*

Reason 12. *Consume alcohol?*

Alcohol depletes the body of many nutrients. If you drink, you need additional B.N.B.B.s. If you have other *Reasons*, the need for B.N.B.B.s gets compounded, e.g. other health problems/treatments.

Reason 13. *Tobacco use?*

Smoking causes depletion of the B.N.B.B.s *per cigarette.*

The only way to know your bases are covered is to make sure you take all the B.N.B.B.s, every day. Take all the B.N.B.B.s everyday, so you leave no holes in your nutritional strategy. And that goes for everyone, not just smokers. *Think!*

If you want to keep smoking that's your business. If you want to make up for some of the damage being done to your body by that nasty habit, well, *that's my business.*

If you want to quit smoking all together you might benefit from reading my book *Too Full To Smoke.* People often describe a complete loss of craving for nicotine when they have the B.N.B.B.s on board. Hypnosis seems to help too.

One of my clients said after taking the B.N.B.B.s consistently, "*I feel too full to smoke.*"

Sometimes what people mistake for cravings of nicotine are actually the brain deficient of the B.N.B.B.s. Once you have enough in your body, the cravings simply go away. Believe it or not, craving nicotine is not because you were born with a shortage of nicotine!

Reason 14. *Marijuana use?*

Marijuana use, regardless where you stand on the subject, depletes the body of Vitamin C, Zinc and other antioxidants. I'm not going to say, *"Don't smoke,"* but if you're going to do it, make sure you make up for the effects it has on the body.

Reason 15. *Air pollution:*

Kind of self-explanatory here. Pollution lowers immunity, increases allergies, reactions and sensitivities in the body and mind.

The B.N.B.B.s offer greater protection to the cellular physiology of the body, strengthening and rebuilding cells, reversing damage done by man-made pollutants and off-setting the likelihood of opportunistic *dis*-ease, as a result of free-radical damage.

Reason 16. *Use laxatives?*

Laxatives, depending on the type used, can interfere with the absorption of nutrients because laxatives tend to speed up and interfere with the process of food passing through the digestive system, giving the nutrition less time to be absorbed. Some laxatives, the common, over-the-counter ones may dump a chemical into the gut, which interferes with absorption as well as directs higher than normal amounts of water to the large intestine, thereby changing the balance of essential electrolytes, which are necessary for the brain and heart to function optimally.

Reason 17. *Fad diets:*

Think it through people! The RDA and DVI% values for nutrition are based on ideal situations where people are consuming 2,000 calories each day and aren't very active. Have you ever heard of anyone doing a weight-loss diet on 2,000 calories a day? No! Dieters aren't getting enough food to get even their very minimum amounts of nutrition-density…within a short time, they are so ravenous for food (due to under-nutrition), that they binge which sort of makes the whole point of withholding food in the first place moot...part of the reason that fast, weight-loss from low calorie/withholding (and low nutrition-density) isn't sustainable for anyone.

If you want to lose weight, until you get enough B.N.B.B.s you'll always have a struggle burning fat, thereby losing healthy weight (lean mass, bone mass, etc.). Any weight you do lose will be short-lived, as the body tries to make up for the mal-nutrition with additional consumption and even more weight gained back due to intense cravings.

Ask me how to do a one-eighty and get on a healthy fat-loss program.

Reason 18. *Over-cooking:*

Vitamins, minerals and especially live enzymes are particularly sensitive to the heat of cooking. Consider vegetables that may not have enough nutrition to begin with, as a result of conventional-farming, nutrient-loss during shipping and processing and what do you imagine you are left with?

The B.N.B.B.s helps make up for gaps in the diet and are processed in a way to keep the 'alive' parts alive. Something cooking, shipping and storage generally do not. The B.N.B.B.s are a sensible way to conveniently get adequate nutrition-density.

Reason 19. *Food processing:* Mineral loss caused by food processing:

Essential minerals (some of the B.N.B.B.s), are some of the things we need to consume in order to utilize the energy available in foods like flour, sugar and rice. Unfortunately, the processing of these basic foods *takes away the very minerals which are needed to digest and assimilate the food themselves,* creating a greater deficit.

In the following examples, look at the amounts of these B.N.B.B.s that are thrown away as a result of the processing the food into junk and fast-energy food and beverage-type edible, consumable products.

Percentage of minerals lost during flour refining:

Chromium† 98%

Cobalt 89%

Manganese 86%

Magnesium* 85% (responsible for 300 different actions).

Sodium 78%

Zinc* 78% (responsible for 300 different actions).

Potassium 77%

Iron 76%

†Chromium is essential for proper functioning of insulin, which is required for fat-loss.

*Magnesium and Zinc alone are each responsible for more than 300 different enzymatic actions required to stay healthy...think of the cascade or chain-of-events that is occurring, at the cellular level, when you aren't getting enough of these B.N.B.B.s each day!

No need to memorize these numbers and percentages. What I would like you to take from these examples is the fact that the very B.N.B.B.s that are removed are the ones that stabilize the chemistry of the body, increasing the rate at which the body *de*-generates into *dis*-ease. Weight gain is a symptom of imbalanced chemistry, as a result of insulin not working properly in the body.

The common factor for people whom want to burn fat is blood sugar that is either too high (insulin-resistance) or the blood sugar swings back and forth (high to low). Nutrition-density (B.N.B.B.s) and stabilizing the blood sugar get the body back in fat-burning mode.

Mineral loss caused by food processing:

	White flour	Sugar refining	Rice polishing
Chromium	98%	95%	92%
Zinc	78%	88%	54%
Manganese	86%	89%	75%

20. *Eat a convenience diet?*

Like most of us, we're on the go and don't always have time to eat right or even have access to what we know we should be eating. The B.N.B.B.s can make up for gaps in our day-to-day habits easily and affordably. *The B.N.B.B.s are not a substitute for Whole-foods, but supplemental to Whole-foods and should be viewed this way.*

For example, when Chromium is deficient in the diet, people experience blood sugar symptoms like low or high blood sugar swings and insulin resistance (Type-2 diabetes). The medical names for these red warning lights are hypoglycemia (low blood sugar), and diabetes (high blood sugar). When we go to the doctor, for either problem, it's likely we will be taught how to exercise and eat better to hopefully manage blood sugar and we may be prescribed a drug(s), which cover up the symptoms of being deficient of the B.N.B.B.s, which prevent the problems to begin with without addressing the underlying problem and have side-effects that cause further *de*-generation of the system and capabilities of the body. But, in a health care system which seems to focus on 'treating' the symptoms, as if they can be separated from the body, some health care professionals have not seemed to understand this underlying cycle, before now, and/or prescribe (synthetic) nutritional supplements which do not nourish the cells the same way (more on this later in the *Choosing Good B.N.B.B.*s chapter).

In addition, the prescription drugs have side-effects, like damage to the circulatory system (heart *dis*-ease, stroke, amputation of the limbs, etc.), and blindness, as well as damage to the internal organs, which then, have to filter out the waste products of the drugs. *Now we are at least four-steps, into the Black-forest,* off the path to optimal health and peak performance. Most people in this scenario end up on more drugs, in an attempt to squelch the symptoms the first set of drugs caused. Drugs do not make up for lack of nutrition-density, resistance-training or cardiovascular exercise conditioning.

Selenium is really important for preventing cancer and 16% of it is removed from flour.

Zinc is essential for the immune system. It's very important for healthy, vital looking skin and 78% of it is removed from flour. Know anyone whom might like to have healthier skin, hair, nails and lips? Or children whom are often sick? Sore throats that go away and then come back again?

Potassium is essential for regulating blood pressure. Know anyone on high blood pressure medication?

People often think of the bones in the spine or arms, legs and hips when there is talk of the need for calcium in the diet. Do you think if the overall bone mass of the body is decreased from lack of nutrition it shows up in the face? It does. Loss of bone mass in the facial bones makes people look older.

Missing from the food-chain?

A few of the trace minerals are actually necessary for *plant* health and resistance. Magnesium, Zinc, Iron, Copper, Calcium, Boron, Manganese, Molybdenum, Cobalt and Chromium, for example, are needed by the plant body *and* human body. But the absence of one element from the soil can cause great health problems, since when it is absent in the soil, as a result of over-farming, it cannot be replaced in fresh produce once the plant has grown.

If inorganic-Cobalt is missing from the soil (due to conventional-farming and over-farming the soil), the plant cannot absorb what is not there to begin with. The plant can't convert the unavailable Inorganic-Cobalt into Organic-Cobalt, to be used by the body…it isn't there! Without Organic-Cobalt, the human body cannot manufacture Vitamin B12 (one of the eight B-Complex group). When we don't have enough B12 our body we can't assimilate Iron properly to make red blood cells to deliver oxygen throughout our body. The body becomes anemic. Anemia causes weakness, fatigue, depression and vulnerability to the *de*-generative *dis*-eases. *Is this making sense?*

Mark Hyman, MD, Says *"In a perfect world, no one would need supplements. But given the stress of our modern life, the poor quality of our food supply, and the high load of toxins on our brains and bodies, most of us need a basic daily supply of the raw materials for all our enzymes and biochemistry to run as designed."*

Chapter Two

What are *your* reasons?

When the body lacks one or more nutritional element(s), the tissue structure of the body is weakened, *i.e., muscles, organs, connective tissue, immune system, reproductive system, etc.*

A reason for this is that B.N.B.B.s combine in the body to form such critical materials as hormones, enzymes, proteins and many other essential building supplies.

For example: If the body is missing Zinc and Chromium (which most junk and fast-energy foods and beverages have zero of), the pancreas cannot properly manufacture and assimilate insulin. The inability of the pancreas to manufacture insulin results in the *de*-generative *dis*-ease known as diabetes. One of the *dis*-eases that used to be reserved for adults that has skyrocketed, in terms of frequency in children, teens and adults under 30-years of age...*in America*...where convenience foods are cheaper than nutritionally-dense food and dietary-supplements are considered, by many to be "extreme" behavior and S.A.D.C.R.A.P. is considered "normal".

When an abundance of the junk and fast-energy food and beverage is consumed regularly, the excessive release of insulin, in response to the refined carbohydrate diet can result in a resistance to the essential benefits of insulin, known as insulin resistance/diabetes, which results in excessive gain of fat...excessive energy stored in the body, but inaccessible for weight-loss and energy production.

The shortage of one mineral may cause more damage in one organ than another. To begin with, the symptoms of the shortage may show up in one part of the body for one person and another part of the body in other people...confusing for a person whom views the body as something to be 'treated' versus maintained. A potassium shortage, for example, will affect every tissue, organ, system and capability of the body, but the signs and outward symptoms (the dashboard warning-light, if you will) will appear in the heart more than any other. This is because potassium acts as a heartbeat regulator. A deficiency of potassium results in irregular heartbeat.

If this happened to you, you could go to the doctor and get an official diagnosis of tachycardia and an excellent prognosis for living an average life, as long as you took the drug that was prescribed to you....*all the while, the not so obvious effects of Potassium deficiency continue, outside your awareness,* because the drug is like a piece of tape that covers up that annoying dashboard warning light...*yes, a generalization.*

Now, if this described a pregnant woman, where would her unborn child be getting her nutrition from if her mom's body does not have enough for mom to begin with?

So, we can see how the body becomes vulnerable to the *de-generative dis*-eases, when the diet is short on some or all of the B.N.B.B.s. Some people start out with higher amounts depending how much mom had (at time of conception). Some people start out with less, especially if mom had less and coped with the feelings of lack of nutrition by supplementing with S.A.D.C.R.A.P. Make sense?

Anything made with white flour has had almost every bit of nutrition stripped away, making the body use its nutritional resources to sort through the food lacking in nutrition, with very little in return. The processing of the food makes the food last longer, so it has a longer shelf-life and profits for the company are more stable and easier to count on. Much of the bread, pastries, candy, chips and TV dinners are all in this category.

I'm not going to tell you to, *"Never eat S.A.D.C.R.A.P."* As a nutrition coach, I suggest people *make the transition slowly.* Anywhere from 4-12 months is reasonable (while building up nutrition-density with the B.N.B.B.s). It takes time to recognize the emotional feelings, of seeming to be deprived, of the things which seem like a reward, but interfere with attainment of fitness goals as well as overall health & wellness. Junk food product consumption is programmed into us by the advertisers of these 'food' products

(S.A.D.C.R.A.P). and compounded by the lack of nutrition-density (B.N.B.B.s). Combine that with, and in combination with, the consumption of low nutrient-density foods, on the brain, and therefore the emotional state we can feel that motivates 'emotional' eating. It takes time to realize just how manipulated we have been to think that the convenience foods are a privilege of modern society. It takes time for the levels of the B.N.B.B.s to build up in the body/brain where cravings for S.A.D.C.R.A.P. disappear completely...a month or two for cravings to completely go away, as long as you maintain the nutrient-density in your brain and body, but that is relatively fast considering people go years without relief from cravings and yo-yo dieting.

A lot of people feel as though they are being punished if they don't 'get' to eat the 'tasty', fast-energy junk...*I used to*. As if putting things in the body, which taste good to malnourished folks, but little by little destroy the immune system is a *privilege*. After all we have worked hard for our money and we can spend it however we want. And it's our body, right?

"Nobody gonna' tell me I ain't have me ice cream!" I hear it all the time...*a symptom of too little nutrition-density in the brain...*and then comes *"...can't figure out why my back hurts all the time!...why my knees hurt?...and the sugar diabetes is gettin' me down!"*

All those things are true. (Did you get that little hint I just threw in there?). *Junk-food only tastes good to people whom don't have enough B.N.B.B.s in their brain and body.*

Junk-food only tastes good to people whom are *under-nourished.*

Junk-food only tastes good to people whom are *under-nourished.*

Once you apply the principles in this book consistently, cravings and a likeness for all the fast-energy stuff goes away. You won't believe how much better you will look and feel. People will be commenting on it, to you.

It reminds me of an anti-drug commercial I used to see on TV. It showed a businessman in a restroom stall snorting cocaine. He was saying to himself, *"I use coke so I can work more, so I can make more money, so I can buy more coke, so I can work more, so I can make more money, so I can buy more coke."* Sounds like insanity, right? That is the very same thing that is going on with processed food in America right now. A lot of addiction and dependency relates to a shrinking of the brain matter, on the front of the brain, which relates to making good decisions for the self.

Only instead of being strung out and emotionally bankrupt, with the inside of the nose burned away, people are experiencing obesity, diabetes, heart *dis*-ease, over-active or under-active immune systems, fatigue and 'un-diagnosable' mystery conditions, such as Syndrome-X at epidemic levels, with no end in sight.

And they are occurring at younger and younger ages. The people whom seem relatively healthy can't figure out why they don't heal or suffer numerous complications, when they have to have general-elective surgery or suffer an unexpected trauma like a fall, or injury like a car accident. Or wonder why a simple thing like a cold or flu bug lasts for weeks. Or why a simple surgery leads to a staph infection that kills 25% of the people whom catch it in the hospital. *"Why won't my back quit hurting!?"*

Think in terms of a savings account:

S.A.D.C.R.A.P. creates an overdrawn health-savings account. Eating fast-food for energy is like borrowing money to place a big bet, losing, then taking out a 'little' loan to place another bet, in hopes you will win enough to repay both loans...*it never works out* because until you supplement with the B.N.B.B.s you simply aren't likely to get ahead of the curve.

When the energy and good stuff is not in the food to begin with, eating and drinking more doesn't create more energy...it creates an overdrawn account that gets worse with time, resulting in symptoms, signs, feelings and other warning lights that there aren't enough B.N.B.B.s circulating and being distributed within the body.

To me, the real bummer is seeing people living from one fast-food-fix to the next, all the while the body is slowly, day-by-day *de*-generating itself into a *dis*-ease. Then one day they have a health problem, thinking 'it just happened' and then go to the doctor to get another chemical to cover up the symptom and then needing more drugs to cover up the symptoms of the drugs. *Way into the "Black-Forest" now.* I know this cycle well because I unwittingly lived it for over 20-years and watched many in my family do the same before me.

Enriched means bankrupt!

Remember seeing the words 'fortified' and 'enriched' on food packages like milk, bread and cereals in the store? Know what it means? It means you've been nutritionally and financially robbed...it's just that you've been told when it's happening.

During the processing of raw food materials, like wheat for example, more than 25-different nutrients and co-factors, which your body has to have, are removed in order to turn the wheat into white flour to make boxed cereals, hamburger buns and pastries. A long, long time ago people knew this. I mean a *lonnnggg* time ago. Clear back in the 1800's people were writing and talking about the same things as I am here. In an attempt to offset the obvious insanity of removing the very ingredients that make it possible for the body to process and utilize the food we eat, the government stepped in and said food processors have to add back *some* of the stuff that was removed.

One time, I watched a program on PBS explaining a lot of the processes of the mass immigration to America, during the late 1800's to early 1900's. One of the schemes that mothers immigrating to America, with their children, were exposed to was that 'officials' at the immigration offices were encouraging mothers to throw away any of their own food they brought with them and begin adopting the 'convenience' of the readily available, yet highly processed dairy and grain snacks, which was actually a scheme to mass market processed foods to new immigrants...to expand the market.

Luckily, each immigrant group brought with them their own cultural foods/recipes, which added immense variety to foods that were available in the U.S. A similar experience was happening when I was born. My mother was told that I shouldn't be nursed or even provided nutritional formula, but rather fed white corn syrup mixed into dairy milk. This led to extensive digestive problems, allergies and poor responding immune system that lasted well into my 20's when I discovered and applied the information, that I'm sharing with you here.

Sooo, food manufacturers add back [four-or-five vitamins] plus some Iron, since they know how to test for blatant deficiencies of Iron. Makes sense, right? And people notice it relatively quickly if they are low of Iron, right? Remove 25, add back 4-or-5, then cover up the symptoms of malnutrition with drugs and call it fortified! *WELCOME to the Black-Forest*, you are welcome to stay as long as you can live because a lot of money will be made from you along the way...*treating the symptoms of purposely withholding the B.N.B.B.s creates!*

Imagine yourself standing on a street corner, in the dead of winter. Someone comes along and robs you of all your possessions including your clothes. As they are running away, they glance back at you for a minute and feel bad you're standing there naked and shivering. So, they give you your socks back. Now *you've been enriched.* You feel better, right?... right?

How can this be?

Every time people begin to learn what the food industry is doing in their factories, consumer advocate groups try to get stronger laws passed about what is legal and what isn't, while food manufacturing lobby groups push to decrease product labeling information, so they can continue to sell minimally nutritious foods which won't spoil sitting on the shelves, which in turn increases the profit for the food producers, since processed foods don't spoil as readily, making profits more predictable.

But because there is so much money at stake, for the food manufacturers of America, the food-producers pay their lobbying politicians to go to war for them. Essentially preventing the public from knowing exactly what they're paying for and consuming until the very latest time. This doesn't only occur in the food industry. We have seen and heard about it with the cigarette companies, the automotive industries with Ford and tires and even asbestos in the automotive brake industry. In 2002 it was leaked to the press that all this time that we have known asbestos to be a known cancer-causing substance, the brake-pad industry has been making the brake pads out of asbestos, for years, without having to notify the public because of a secret legal settlement. Meaning all these years, brake repair specialists and everyone else whom is ever around moving automobiles has been unknowingly exposed to asbestos in the air we all breathe. On January 14, 2003, I read in the Seattle newspapers that the major automotive manufacturers were trying to get out of any liability for asbestos for the brake pads they installed on all their autos, for all the years this has been going on.

The establishment of lobby groups is a double-edged sword. Lobbyists prevent unfair treatment of groups of people with like interests. As a massage therapist, I was part of an association which helps set standards and promote the medical benefits of massage therapy and to familiarize state legislators with the legitimate uses of massage therapy.

So, to make a long story short, we now have standard food labels with *some* nutrition facts, on the label. Most food produced and sold in the United States have this on the packaging to help us make health-based decisions. If you want the benefits I refer to throughout this book, you may want to familiarize yourself with it, but do research beyond food labels to make sure you get enough B.N.B.B.s.

Food labels:

Here, is what food labels tell us: Of the more than 25-different nutrients we need, the government regulation says only a few of the nutrients need be listed/shown. And, of the four listed on nutritional labels, (Vitamins A, C, plus the minerals Iron and calcium), **they don't have to be in the food**, *they just have to tell us they aren't in the food!* Which in itself implies each of us is going to know how to make up the nutritional difference for what we didn't get from foods, as well as have a strategy for getting the B.N.B.B.s somewhere else…yet, then we're told we don't need to supplement…*whaaaat?!*

Take the example on the next page. Read down the label. Notice four-nutrients are listed. Vitamins A & C, Calcium and Iron are listed, but in the quantity of zero.

This example happens to be some Swedish, whole-grain crackers. Notice the amounts of nutrients listed:

Nutrition Facts:

Serving Size: 1 slice (11 g)

Servings Per Container: about 23

Amount Per Serving

Calories 35 Calories from fat 0%

Daily Value:

Total Fat 0g 0%

Saturated Fat 0g 0%

Polyunsaturated Fat 0g 0%

Monounsaturated Fat 0g 0%

Cholesterol 0g 0%

Sodium 45mg 2%

Total Carbohydrates 9g 3%

Dietary Fiber 2g 6 %

Sugars 0 grams

Protein

Vitamin A 0%

Vitamin C 0%

Calcium 0%

Iron 2%

Isn't it S.A.D.?

Studies show that today, even with our 'enriched food', over 92% of Americans are deficient in one-or-more vitamins. There's tons of similar studies that show higher or lower percentages...*just look.*

That doesn't mean they are receiving less than the amount they need for optimal health. That means they receive less than the MINIMUM amount necessary to prevent deficiency *dis*-eases...a gradual breaking-down of the body, from the inside out. The Standard American Diet, or S.A.D., for short, may support mediocre health for a while, but it won't build optimal health or prevent *de*-generative *dis*-ease(s) and by itself doesn't come close to providing enough nutrition-density for fitness, fat loss and/or athletics.

Without enough nutrition-density, the body inevitably begins breaking down. Most people don't understand the role of vitamins and minerals, in their body, nor the direct correlation between how they feel and how much nutrition has stored up in their body. I certainly didn't when I finished various training courses. What most people don't realize is the same thing I was unaware of when I first started practicing: *The real reason our food supply must be 'enriched' is because it is has be so processed that it is 'impoverished' to start with.*

In a study from the *Journal of the American College of Nutrition,* researchers found that 6% of those people tested had serious Vitamin C deficiency and 30% were borderline low. A report in the journal *Pediatrics* found obesity and malnutrition coexisting. Obese, overfed, and undernourished children with cognitive disorders were found to have scurvy and severe Vitamin D deficiency, also known as rickets. These deficiencies damage our children's bodies and brains. You never think of an overweight person as malnourished, but they are!..*overfed and under-nourished*....meaning they are getting enough calories to gain fat (unhealthy insulin-resistance), but inadequate nutrition to release the fat for energy (healthy insulin-sensitivity).

A United States Department of Agriculture survey showed that 37% of Americans don't get enough Vitamin C, 70% not enough Vitamin E, almost 75% don't get enough Zinc, and 40% don't get enough Iron. Based on what I have experienced and seen with others over the decades, I would say 100% of us don't have enough of the basic nutrients as much as we need to.

The website nutrition.gov says, *"If you are already eating the recommended amount of a nutrient, you may not get any further health benefit from taking a supplement."* This sort of circular logic can interfere with people's ability to make concrete decisions for themselves and feel good about it. **Why would any health professional suggest someone is getting enough nutrition, but not demonstrate how to test if they actually are getting enough nutrition? (Leaving it to chance!).**

https://www.nutrition.gov/dietary-supplements/questions-ask-taking-vitamin-and-mineral-supplements

Dr. Robert Heaney, one of the world's leading Vitamin D researchers, in a recent groundbreaking editorial in *The American Journal of Clinical Nutrition,* about the delayed (yet very serious) consequences of taking less than the optimal amounts of nutrients for life, said, *"...because the current [vitamin] recommendations are based on the prevention of the [deficiency] disease only, they can no longer be said to be biologically defensible. The pre-agricultural human diet...may well be a better starting point for policy. The burden of proof should fall on those whom say that these more natural conditions are not needed and that lower intakes [of nutrients] are safe."*

In other words, as each generation gets less and less nutrition, than generation is used to set the standard for the next generation...how does that make any sense? Essentially, instead of figuring out what the body needs and sticking to it (which would increase costs for the food manufacturers, distributors and government agencies), standards for nutrition are being set based on *how little humans can get by with...*rather than how much nutrition-density we need, which is the opposite standard used to keep domestic farm animals healthy. If nutrition standards are set higher, manufacturers would make less profit and subsequently place pressure on government to once again lower the standards, which increases cost of medical care to consumer and tax payers. The only option is for each consumer to make sure they get enough nutrition-density based on their goals, lifestyle, eating habits, goals, level of health and so forth. If you don't take it on, no one else will do it for you. Health truly is a personal responsibility. Even if a doctor told me to take the B.N.B.B.s I still have to get them and take them myself as most insurance doesn't cover nutrition.

Does it make any sense at all for health professionals who aren't getting enough nutrition to make recommendations to their patients?

Dr. Heaney went on to say, *"In today's world, everyone needs a basic multivitamin and mineral supplement. The research is overwhelming on this point. My own experience as a practitioner corresponds to what the research tells us. I have tested for vitamin and nutrient deficiencies in thousands-of-patients and found that by correcting them people feel better, improve their mood, mental sharpness, memory and ability to focus, as well as have more energy, resolve chronic health complaints or conditions and even lose weight. Taking supplements also helps prevent disease. The basic vitamin recommendations outlined below include nutrients that form the backbone for proper optimal biological function, robust health, and healthy aging. These nutrients work as a team and the basic workhorse team outlined below should be taken by everyone."*

An article was published in the *Journal of the American Medical Association*, entitled *Whom takes dietary-supplements, and why? February 14, 2013*

Approximate percentage of adults under and over age 50 **using dietary-supplements**, NHANES Surveys, 1972-2006:

NHANES I: 1971-1974: Adults younger than 50 (22%). Adults older than 50 (27%).

NHANES II: 1976-1980: Adults younger than 50 (33%). Adults older than 50 (39%).

NHANES III: 1988-1994: Adults younger than 50 (40%). Adults older than 50 (46%).

NHANES 1999-2000: Adults younger than 50 (45%) . Adults older than 50 (60%).

NHANES 2003-2006: Adults younger than 50 (45%). Adults older than 50 (67%).

NHANES data from the Council For Responsible Nutrition:

• 49% of adults used a supplement of some kind of supplements in the prior 30 days: 54% of women, 43% of men.

• Supplement use increased with age: 34% aged 20-39, 50% age 40-59, and 67% over age 60.

• Non-Hispanic whites use more supplements (54%) than Non-Hispanic blacks (38%) or Hispanics (33%).

• Supplement use is greater in 'never' (51%) or 'former' (59%) smokers compared to current smokers (30%-36%).

• Supplement use is much more common in those with health insurance (53%) than those without (31%).

• Supplement use parallels reported exercise, from 'low' (43%) to 'moderate' (54%) to 'high' (56%).

• Supplement use was higher among those that reported 'excellent' or 'very good' health (55%) versus 'good' (47%) or fair/poor (44%).

Wealthier and healthier supplement users tend to be a higher percentage than non-users. It's the 'healthy user' effect which shows up throughout epidemiological studies.

https://sciencebasedmedicine.org/whom-takes-dietary-supplements-and-why/

Reasons people take dietary-supplements (average age older than 20-years) 2007-2010:

Anemia - 5%.

Eye health - 4%.

Weight-loss - 3%.

Skin health - 5%.

Bone health - 25%.

Mental health - 5%.

Improved sleep - 1%.

To stay healthy - 33%.

Enhanced energy - 11%.

Supplement the diet - 22%.

Healthy hair and nails - 1%.

Prevent health problems - 20%.

To improve overall health - 45%.

Heart health/lower cholesterol - 15%.

Boost immunity/prevent colds - 15%.

Healthier joints/prevent arthritis - 12%.

* Dietary-supplement sales in the United States has reached $30 billion (2011).

A related survey, also recently published in *JAMA Internal Medicine, Users' Views of Dietary-supplements,* gives additional insight to the NHANES survey on motivations for use of supplements. Blendon and colleagues at the Harvard School of Public Health conducted a telephone survey of 1,579 people aged 18 or older. This survey asked specifically about dietary-supplements and identified 584 supplement users. 38% reported taking any supplement in the past two-years, and 13% reported taking a supplement regularly, which appears in the ballpark of the NHANES study. Fish oil/Omega-3 oils were the most common consumed (again, consistent with NHANES) with 24% consuming the product in the past two-years. Reasons reported for taking supplements included:

● To feel better - 41%.

● Digestive issues - 28%.

● Lower cholesterol - 21%.

● To boost your immune system - 36%.

● To improve your overall energy levels - 41%.

Over 80% reported it was important to have access to supplements. Interestingly, users were asked how government-sponsored efficacy studies would influence their decision to take a supplement. Amazingly, only 25% of users said they would stop using a supplement if it was evaluated to be ineffective. Also, interesting: 36% of supplement users had not told their physician about their supplement use, while 31% reported a physician or nurse had recommended their supplement use.

A third study showed similar results: From the Military Nutrition Division of the US Army, it's entitled *Confidence in the efficacy and safety of dietary-supplements among United States active duty army personnel* and was published in *BMC Complementary and Alternative Medicine* in 2012. This was a survey of 990 soldiers in 2006-07 at 11 military bases that focused on motivations, not specific supplements taken.

A dietician or other health professional administered the questionnaire directly and asked for usage of supplements as defined by DSHEA. The sample group was mainly male (87%), white (70%), and young (41% were aged 18-24). Just over 1/2 (53%) reported using supplements, at least once per week, during the prior 6 weeks. Usage was observed to be highest among those older in age, better educated, and holding higher ranks, and reporting good/excellent health.

2/3 (67%) of all participants were somewhat confident or extremely/very confident in the efficacy of supplements, which increased to 86% among users. The majority of non-users (62% were not at all confident in supplement efficacy). Those whom reported excellent fitness or dietary habits were much more likely to be very/extremely confident in supplement efficacy.

In other words, the people whom consistently take dietary-supplements (B.N.B.B.s) are confident they work while the people whom do not take them are not confident they work! LOL.

AIDS and vitamins?

An article in The New York Times on July 1, 2004 entitled *Daily Vitamin Can Thwart AIDS Progress, Study Says*, talked about the benefits of dietary-supplements used in combination with AIDS drugs.

Comments within the article included, *"A daily multivitamin pill can delay the progress of AIDS in HIV infected...according to a study done at Harvard University and published in The NEW England Journal of Medicine...$15 worth of vitamins given over the course of a year can lengthen the life..,"* This is exciting because it costs literally pennies and can ward off the time of treatment with toxic and expensive drugs have to be started, said Dr. Richard G. Marlink, whom helps ran treatment programs in six African countries as Director of the Harvard AIDS Institute said, *"... the study would prompt him to recommend vitamins to his patients."*

"The supplements do not attack the virus, but enhance the body's own immune system, allowing it to do so." (Remember, I said the immune system is made of and relies on the B.N.B.B.s to be able to do their jobs?).

"...the vitamins are quite easy to mass produce," said its lead author Wafale W. Fawzi, a professor of nutrition and epidemiology at Harvard. They contained about [three times the recommended daily allowance] of Vitamin E, and six-to-ten times the amount of Vitamin C and B-Complex.

"...Tanzania study found that 30% fewer whom received the Multi-vitamin died or progressed to full AIDS during the study."

"...the counts of the immune cells the virus attacks stayed somewhat higher in the group that took the Multi-vitamins...also, had fewer incidents of thrush, throat ulcers, inflamed gums, nausea, rashes, fatigue and other debilitating." Many researchers noticed that vitamin-deficient patients sickened faster. Three-years ago Dr. Andrew Thomkins at the Institute of Child Health in London, gave Multi-vitamins to 481 HIV-infected men and women in Thailand *and he said, "...the group taking vitamins had significantly lower mortality, especially among those whom their immune systems were weakest."*

"...those whom benefited from the vitamins did so "regardless whether they were* [considered] *undernourished or not," Dr. Fawzi said.

AMA reverses its recommendations:

In 2002, The American Medical Association reversed its recommendations in relation to taking dietary-supplements. *About-Face: JAMA recommends Multi-vitamins:*

Studies indicate that everybody, regardless of age or health status, should take a daily Multivitamin/mineral.

"After 20-years, the Journal of the American Medical Association has completely reversed its policy and is now

encouraging all adults to take at least one Multi-vitamin per day. A landmark article published in the journal announced that, "...all adults should take vitamin supplements to prevent chronic diseases.""

"Most people do not consume an optimal amount of all vitamins, by diet alone. It appears prudent for all adults to take vitamin supplements," state the articles by Robert H. Fletcher, MD, MSc, and Kathleen M. Fairfield, MD, Dr.PH, both affiliated with Harvard Medical School. The physicians reviewed studies published between 1966 and 2002 that investigate the links between vitamin intake and *dis*-eases such as cancer, osteoporosis, and coronary heart *dis*-ease.

A [large proportion of the population is at increased risk due to low vitamin levels]. The high prevalence of these *dis*-eases indicates the standard diet in the U.S. fails to provide sufficient amounts of the vitamins studied. The authors examined the following nutrients: Vitamins A, B6, B12, C, D, E, and K, Folate, and the carotenoids including Alpha-and Beta-carotene, Beta-Cryptoxanthin, Lycopene, Lutein, and Zeaxanthin.

They noted the association of low intakes of the B-vitamins with elevated homocysteine levels and the increased risk of coronary heart *dis*-ease; of low Folate with neural tube defects, coronary heart *dis*-ease, breast cancer, and colorectal cancer; of Vitamin B6 deficiency with cheilosis, stomatitis, central nervous system effects, and neuropathy; of low B12 with macrocytic anemia and neurologic abnormalities; of low levels of Vitamin E with prostate cancer; of low levels of various carotenoids with breast, prostate, and lung cancer; of low Vitamin D with secondary hyperparathyroidism, bone loss, osteoporosis, and increased fracture risk; of low Vitamin C with cancer; of low Vitamin A with vision disorders and decreased immune function; and of low Vitamin K with blood clotting disorders and with increased fracture risk.

Drs. Fletcher and Fairfield recommend that [everybody, regardless of age or health status, take a daily multivitamin/mineral].

The physicians go on to suggest that vegans, whom may not get enough Vitamins D and B12, also need to take a Multi-vitamin.

In addition, as people age, they become less able to absorb vitamins and minerals from their diet and should take a Multi-vitamin, the physicians said. Reference: *Journal of the American Medical Association,* 2002; 287:3116-26, 3127-29.

Chapter Three

Getting it?

Reason 21. Have food or environmental allergies?

I used to! When the body is deficient of the B.N.B.B.s the integrity of the cells of the body is sub-par. In other words, the walls of the cells aren't as strong and flexible as they are capable of being. Things get inside the cell that shouldn't and things that should be kept in the cell slip out making the energy production and storage, immune-response and separation between the different types of cells seem to become 'confused and compromised'. The net result is allergic-type reactions, as the body tries to prevent things from getting worse.

In my life, I seemed to be 'allergic' (for lack of better term) to chocolate (made my nose bleed) tomato products like pizza and spaghetti sauce (made my face itch like crazy for a couple days after consumption) most vegetables (gave me diarrhea) as well as seasonal hay-fever type allergies that about drove me out of my mind (severe), from May through October, each year. I kept increasing the amount of OTC medications, as well as some prescriptions, which worked for a while, then stopped working.

Once I consistently got the B.N.B.B.s in my body, the 'allergies' to foods 'mysteriously' went away. Today, the only limitations to my diet are personal preferences. As far as the hay-fever, all of the symptoms have improved. I don't know if they would work for everyone as well as they worked for me, but there's no risk in finding out. I don't recommend 'treating' symptoms, but rather put nutrition in the body, as a course of maintenance and let nature take over from there. The body will use what it needs, if the quality of the B.N.B.B.s is high enough, for you.

People whom know about that kind of stuff describe that benefit as healthier/stronger mast-cells, which when properly developed, are less likely to release histamines prematurely or contribute to allergic symptoms (allergies).

Reason 22. Inconsistent crop nutrition levels:

Folks whom practice 'medicinal' or 'theory-based nutrition' rely heavily on databases, which are supposed to provide nutritional information about what we eat. Problem? These professionals treat the information as holy in that they behave as if the food tested and listed in their database is the same food that you and I eat on a daily basis, today...*it's not.* If that weren't enough, they routinely say things like, *"Well, if you're eating these foods and you are 'healthy' you 'should' have a 'balanced' diet and so you 'probably' don't need vitamin supplements...you likely get what you need from food."* Hear and see the problems within that statement?

The problems I have with that is that, once again, they behave as if what is in their text books or computer databases is what is really going into the body...often (it's how they wish things were happening), so their treatment of their patients would match what their textbook insists.

Using the word 'should' leaves a lot of gaps between what our bodies require nutritionally and what we actually do in daily-habit, because it isn't definitive. It implies you're healthy when they don't know your nutritional status. Also, that they use words like 'balanced' as if you and I know what balanced means to a nutritionist or that it means the same thing to both of us or that everyone agrees on what 'balanced' means...there's a hundred or more models of eating that each person insists is correct and that doesn't even take cultural, regional or religious standards into account. No matter what style you choose to follow, you still have to get enough B.N.B.B.s. That statement demonstrates a bias that leaves too much room for the public to make choices assuming that in general they are getting 'enough' nutrition-density, without actually knowing it to be true. And in reality, many studies show that the majority of the population is missing key nutrients, on a daily basis, for months and years at a time, without acknowledging the correlation with the most common *dis*-eases.

In addition, since the mass immigration to America in the late 1800's and people were coming from all over the world with many, many models of eating ...everyone knows America is made up of 60+ different nationalities...*why only one government food guide pyramid?*

Think about it!..regardless of the food model, if it doesn't assure enough nutrition-density (B.N.B.B.s/amount of vitamins, minerals, enzymes, etc.), it isn't likely to provide any noticeable, measurable improvement in how you feel or look, let alone improvement in blood chemistry, lab results.

A person might lose 'weight' by decreasing calories, but without adequate nutrition-density/B.N.B.B.s, cravings are likely and sustaining the weight-loss versus burning fat and gaining healthy lean tissue beyond three-months is not likely at all...hence, short-term success followed by intense cravings, binging and gaining more weight back than was lost.

The foods that Farmer Joe grows in California is not going to have the same soil conditions as Farmer Jane in Washington, a field in the Midwest, nor from one field to the next let alone county or region. Yet, nutritional data bases that dieticians tend to use behave as if all vegetables and fruits have the same amount of nutrients across-the-board...*they do not.* When they run into patients whom don't seem to respond to their mediocre nutrition recommendations, they consider the patient the anomaly rather than the fact that their 'database' is off. I've had many clients report this sequence.

The nutritional data bases are based on the health of the soil in the 1930's.

The Associated Press reported, on January 7, 2001, that broccoli contains a cancer fighting chemical known as Glucocoraphanin. But, the Department of Agriculture studied 71-types of broccoli and found a 30-fold difference, in the amounts of the cancer fighting chemical. Farmers and consumers can't tell the difference between the types of broccoli, without a laboratory test. *"Nearly everything is highly variable in plants,"* says Paul Talalay, a specialist in cancer prevention at the Johns Hopkins University Medical Center.

The food tested to set the standards is not the food we eat. Dr. Michael Colgan, author of *Your Personal Vitamin Profile* tested various oranges from local markets. He found the content of Vitamin C varied from 0 milligrams up to 180 milligrams. Every piece of food is different. What follows is another example:

Eating vegetables causes high blood pressure?

Non Certified-Organically Grown (conventionally-farmed), supermarket produce appears to be giving toady's Americans more salt and less nutrition than generally recognized. In 1989, Nutrient Testing Laboratories, Ltd., of Babylon, New York ran mineral analysis tests on commercial produce from various regions around the U.S.

The results?...well, I'll let you interpret what they mean and how eating your 5-9 servings of produce a day could affect the number of people with heart *dis*-ease today (heart *dis*-ease being one of the top-two killers in America).

The results clearly showed dissimilarity in nutrient content according to soils of different regions. Sodium levels reflecting artificial fertilizer use, were particularly high in all commercially/conventionally grown produce tested.

Nutrient Testing Laboratories, Ltd. (NTL), measured the mineral content of the following produce items:

■ Apples

■ Broccoli

■ Carrots

■ Celery

■ Green peppers

- Peas

- Potatoes

- Red beets

- Spinach

- String beans and

- Tomatoes

All produce was purchased from grocery stores in California, Colorado, Florida, Massachusetts, and New York. NTL's intent was to find out if there were any mineral imbalances, in the soil, in which these foods were grown.

First, they analyzed the foods for their content of 13-minerals. Then they compared how many parts-per-million of the minerals, in a serving size of 3½ ounces, in raw form of each food.

Based on the data, NTL reported that mineral content in each food varied widely from region to region.

For example:

- Colorado's spinach had 5-times more Iron than Florida's spinach.

- Florida's tomatoes had 18-times more Calcium than Massachusetts tomatoes.

- There was 3-times more Phosphorus in California potatoes than New York potatoes.

While some of the food samples contained **[no amount of certain 'essential-for-basic-health' minerals]** all 11-foods contained more salt than previously recorded and more salt than food content data bases, books and food packaging labels represented, which Registered dieticians use to provide nutrition information about nutritional requirements.

In order to compare these results with changes in the quality of food over time, NTL used the H. J. Heinz nutrition chart from 1949, which is considered one of the definitive charts (today), for learning how much nutrition is supposed to be in the food we eat and the kind of information nutritionists and dieticians use to design nutrition programs for healthy and unhealthy people. As a result, *NTL discovered that the salt content of each food had increased substantially, over the last 40-years, as salt-based fertilizer use increased.*

The recent elevation in salt, NTL reported, is likely due to commercial produce farmers' overuse of inorganic-fertilizer, which is highly concentrated forms of inorganic-salt...the most common fertilizer used in conventional-farming to make the plants grow and look healthy [*even when they don't have any nutrition-density, within them].* That is just one-way plants receive only what the farmers give them as supplemental growth factors, as the soil is depleted and demolished through unnatural/conventional-farming practices, which leave the sold void of essential nutritional components, which the body requires to remain healthy.

Putting food in mouth, chewing, drinking and swallowing does not mean you are absorbing or able to utilize the good stuff to get the benefits you want most. It just means you're going through the motions. The amount, of calories you eat does not mean you're getting enough of the B.N.B.B.s either. At one point I was eating over 6,000 calories a day and I was far from healthy, in fact my body fat was 4% and the Registered Dietician I visited insisted all I needed to do was, *"...eat my three-meals-a-day and make sure I get vegetables."* Studies done on Olympic Athletes demonstrated the same kinds of things. Thousands-of-calories-a-day do not assure adequate nutrition-density getting into the cells of the body where they can do good, especially when they aren't there to begin with. As activity level increases, so do nutritional-density requirements.

Fruits and vegetables are only as good as the soil in which they are grown:

In general, nutrients pass from the soil to the plant to our body only when they are present in the soil to begin with...*makes sense right?*

Around World War II large scale commercial farmers were persuaded by the chemical companies that they didn't need to give the farmland time to recover, between each crop. The chemicals that were used so heavily to make bombs and explosives make the plants grow bigger and faster, regardless of the soil condition and nutrient levels within the soil. By applying the synthetic chemicals to the land, plants are forced to grow even without the nutrients that are absolutely essential to our health. The farmers were taught that people will buy the produce, if it *appears* good on the outside.

You see, all the nutrients that people and animals depend on for good health are not necessarily necessary for the plants themselves to grow big and hearty. So, there is very little incentive for Non Certified-Organic farmers to rotate the types of crops, allowing the land to recover between harvests.

The same materials which were surplus after the bomb making efforts of World War II, are what we know as phosphate-based fertilizers, used on Non Certified-Organic crops, since the 1940's and even today (Conventional-farming). These bind with some minerals, keeping them in the ground, making them unavailable to the plants and making them unavailable to people whom eat those crops.

Non Certified-Organic farming uses synthetic (non-nutritive), fertilizer (nitrogen, phosphate and potassium), and pesticides and growth hormones to force the plants to grow, regardless of the amount of nutrition in the plants. That is part of the reason why the oranges that Dr. Michael Colgan tested had from zero milligrams to 180 milligrams of Vitamin C in them. With the use of chemicals and specialized plant breeding, farmers produce fabulous looking produce that can be void of the nutrients that are essential for us to look, feel and perform our best.

Then the food is picked too early, stored, shipped, stored, shipped, stored, sold, cooked, canned, processed and potentially frozen. And what is left our digestive system has to sort through to find anything worth building a healthy cell out of. *And we wonder why we do not have enough energy or bone mass?*

A Tacoma, Washington Newspaper, December 6, 2000, reported that in the apple industry, especially in Yakima, Washington growers are rewarded for the reddest, biggest and best [looking] fruit.

40-years ago, as a little boy, I visited my cousins in Yakima in the heart of apple country. My dad, my cousin and I went on a little adventure to what was the beginning of cold storage and cross-breeding that made apples and other produce last for years, without spoiling after being picked from the tree. We went to a really large building. Bigger than a football field and five-stories tall, the whole interior being a large refrigerator. The special cross-breeding of the fruit makes it appear good on the outside. Then the apples are washed and coated with fungicide-containing wax and put into refrigeration for up to two-years, before they show up on the store shelves, so farmers can stockpile massive amounts of fruit in hopes of increasing profit and predicting profit throughout the year. And that is why the red delicious apples are often so mushy and pulpy inside. They were not that way before people messed around with the genetic makeup of the fruit.

When I worked in a grocery store produce department some kids had a food fight with apples after hours. One of the apples landed atop the produce cooler some eight-feet above the floor. I was curious how long it would take for it to begin to decompose. Five-months later it still hadn't begun to decompose.

In the food industry, there is massive competition to wipe out the types of produce created by nature and replace them with genetically modified forms that can be patented and owned by the two-percent of the population, whom intend to control the entire food industry. That way, any time a farmer grows a certain type of fruit or vegetable, they have to pay a licensing fee so the company that holds the patent makes money from every piece of food sold. In essence, food conglomerates are attempting to control the entire Earth's food production, with little regard for what's best for our health. That is exactly what has happened in the apple industry.

Harvard Women's Health Watch, January 2013, Published an article entitled, *Dietary-supplements: Do they help or hurt? ...*What you need to know before taking a vitamin or mineral supplement:

"The average American diet leaves a lot to be desired. Research finds our plates lacking in a number of essential nutrients, including Calcium, Potassium, Magnesium, and Vitamins A, C, and D. It's no wonder that more than 1/2 of us open a supplement bottle to get the nutrition we need. Many of us take supplements, not just to make up for what we're missing, but also because we hope to give ourselves an extra health boost—a preventive buffer to ward off disease."

Mayo Clinic Says: *"Dietary-supplements also may be appropriate if you...":*

● Don't obtain 2-to-3 servings of fish, per week.

● Don't eat well or consume less than 1,600 calories a day.

● Are a vegan or a vegetarian, whom eats a limited variety of foods.

● Are a woman whom experiences heavy bleeding during your menstrual period.

● Have a medical condition that affects how your body absorbs or uses nutrients, such as chronic diarrhea, food allergies, food intolerance, or a disease of the liver, gallbladder, intestines or pancreas.

• Have had surgery on your digestive tract and are not able to digest and absorb nutrients properly.

So, you can see and hear that by comparing all the different subgroups of people that health experts and organizations say need to supplement, there's actually very *few people whom aren't in at least one of the groups recommended to take dietary-supplements.*

If you're like I was, (with multiple health concerns: allergies, digestive problems, bleeding, picky eater, travel a lot), you may belong to more than one group, compounding the need to supplement your Whole-foods with B.N.B.B.s.

FoodAmerica.org reported on these groups of people:

Seniors:

• More than 5-million senior citizens, age 60 and older face hunger. Seniors face a number of unique medical and mobility challenges that put them at a greater risk of hunger. After a lifetime of hard work, many find themselves struggling with health issues on fixed incomes. Many of these individuals are forced to choose between paying for groceries and buying medicine, so their nutritional intake inevitably suffers.

Feeding America addresses the unique challenges of senior hunger through interventions that take into account the health status, medication needs, transportation, physical limitations and dietary restrictions of older Americans. As the proportion of people over the age of 60 continues to grow, *Feeding America* continues to develop innovative initiatives to get more food to more seniors in need.

• In addition to the senior population, evidence shows that older adults whom are slightly younger – including those in their 50s – may be particularly vulnerable to certain health and nutrition challenges (at higher rates than older seniors).

• 7-million individuals, served by *Feeding America* each year are seniors age 60 or older.

- Additionally, the network also serves nearly 6-million "older adults" ages 50-59.

- More than 33% of client households have at least one member whom is age 60 or older.

- 63% of client households, with seniors, report making choices between paying for food and paying for medicine/medical care.

- 2-in-5 (41%) client households with an adult age 50 and older have at least one member with diabetes, and more than 2/3 (70%) of client households with an older adult have at least one member, whom has high blood pressure. These rates increase with age. However, among older adult clients, those whom are younger report significant health challenges. 59% of those ages 50-to-64 described their own health as fair or poor, a higher rate than that of seniors ages 65% to 74% (53%) and age 75 and older (51%).

Among African-Americans:

While hunger has no boundaries, it does impact some communities more than others.

- African Americans are more likely to suffer from food insecurity as their white, Non-Hispanic counterparts.

- They are disproportionately affected by unemployment and poverty as well.

Among Mexican-Americans:

- Among all *Feeding America* clients, 20% are Latino. Nearly 1-in-6 Latinos in America are served by the *Feeding America Network.*

- More than 1-in-5 (22%) Latino households are food insecure compared to just 1 in 10 (11 %) of Caucasian households and 1-in-7 (14%) households, overall.

Rural Hunger Facts:

• 15% of rural households are food insecure, or an estimated 2.8 million households. In Montana, 31% of children are food insecure, never knowing where their next meal will come from.

• 50% of counties with the highest rates of food insecurity (those in the top 10%), are in rural areas. Rural areas also account for 64% of counties with the highest rates of child food insecurity. For sake of comparison, 42% of all counties are rural. In contrast, 26% of counties with the highest rates of food insecurity are metropolitan, as are 15% of counties with the highest rates of child food insecurity. 37% of all counties are metropolitan.

Rural Poverty Facts:

• 7.4 million Americans (16.7%) living in rural areas live below the federal poverty line.

• Compared to all regions, the South continues to have the highest poverty rate among people in families living in rural areas (15.3%).

• 47% of people in families, with a single female head-of-household living in rural areas, were poor in 2015, as compared to 35% in the suburbs.

So, how can they say most people don't need supplemental B.N.B.B.s?

Chapter Four

"Sov...you won't believe what happened!"

Louise Light, MS, ED.D., former USDA Director of Dietary Guidance and Nutrition Research and author of *Fatally Flawed Food Guide* (2004) and *What to Eat* (2006), whom developed the eating guide that became what we know as The Food Guide Pyramid. Carefully reviewing the research on nutrient recommendations, *dis*-ease prevention, documented dietary shortfalls and major health problems of the population and submitted the final version of The Food Guide to the Secretary of Agriculture.

When the revised edition came back to Luise and the group, they were shocked that it was changed so much that it hardly resembled what Luise's research and recommendations demonstrated.

Later, she found out that the changes were made to win over acceptance from the food manufacturing industry (versus protecting consumers)...those whom manufacture, advertise, promote, market food products to the public and profit from making food cheaper, more shelf-stable and consequently less nutritionally-dense...*to avoid the onslaught of offense by the lobbyists, for the food manufacturing industry.*

The wording of the guidelines, were so changed to emphasize and influence the public's ideas and perceptions of the processed foods over whole-foods, because the food industry advocates feared lost profits if Luises' research results surfaced, within government nutrition recommendations. Servings of wheat were exaggerated to please the wheat growers profit plans. The color of fats on the proposed guidelines (for the public to interpret) was changed from red to purple because the beef ranchers knew that consumers could unconsciously see the connection between red-meat and high blood cholesterol levels and so on.

Whom says we are not getting the nutrition we need?

Light's nutrition research team suggested 5-9 servings of fruits and vegetables each day, taking into consideration how much one needs to eat to get the minimum amount of nutrition-density, but and it was reduced to 2-3 servings per day, to appear more politically-correct.

The suggestion of 3-4 servings of carbohydrate (considering calories rather than amount of nutrition-density) were altered to 6-to-11 servings, in order to boost sales of corn and wheat. Wording like *"eat less"* was changed to *"avoid too much"* as if consumers, or doctors for that matter, would know what *"avoid too much"* means. In my writing and teachings I call this being 'generally specific', in that the wording is presented to make the 'experts' seem like they gave you some powerful, practical information, but in reality the wording is non-committal and designed this way so that they can seem to be providing the public with critical information (as advocates for consumers) when in reality they word things this way, so that they can continue to be hired by the food manufacturers, but perceived as protecting the public...*politically-correct double-talk.*

Again, language I refer to as 'generally specific'. In other words, consumers, whom use the language think they are doing the right things, yet the statistics for health of the nation demonstrates otherwise. Luise Light has her own books available on Amazon.

Luise vehemently opposed the final version of The Food Guide Pyramid (yet, to her surprise, she was the only one whom opposed it). In 1980 Luise believed that if her recommendations were not integrated for public use, diabetes and obesity would reach epidemic proportions...*and they have haven't they!* On March 7, 2017 it was reported on NBC News that (lack of nutrition has now exceeded tobacco use as the highest risk for heart *dis*-ease, stroke and diabetes). *More on this later.*

In other words, the United States Department of Agriculture has made it easy for food producers to *control the messages* Americans get, as far as what is considered/promoted as healthy, placing profits ahead of American-health. Often, the food producer executives go on to become leaders, within the Department of Agriculture itself, paving the way for all their food-producing buddies…*and the beat goes on.*

Reason 23. To gain strength:

For the beginner, any amount of consistent and proper strength training should produce some improvement in muscular strength, regardless of age.

The point here to take note of is that everyone, whether a weekend warrior or professional athlete, will reach plateaus in their training regime at various points in their training. In other words, the body will only adapt to a certain point and then progress slows or halts until the exercises are changed, up to create new stimulus for the hormone and nervous systems. For the beginner, often the greatest gains in strength come in the first eight-weeks. The building up phase is called anabolic or 'building up'. Meaning, the body has the nutritional resources to adapt to the stress of exercise by getting stronger and more resilient to injury. The catabolic phase being a 'breaking down' of the body, in that the exercise places stress on the body, but without adequate nutritional resources, the systems and capabilities of the body break down faster than they can build up, which of course leads to things like sprains, strains, tendonitis and bone problems like stress fractures and being more vulnerable to viral and bacterial infections/colds/flu. **Low back pain and knee pain being two of the most common complaints.**

A lot of people think that lifting weights is what makes the body get stronger. That's partially true, in that without the activity/stimulus the muscles wouldn't adapt by getting stronger. In reality, when we lift weights the weight-lifting/resistance-training acts as "stimulus" to the nervous and hormone systems, which then combine the nutritional resources, which (should be) [consistently] on board, prior to exercise. The net result being stronger, more resilient muscles. Without adequate B.N.B.B.s the body can't fully carry out the signals for the nervous and hormone systems.

Without optimizing the nutritional surplus, the body will not get as strong in the initial eight-weeks, and additionally will likely suffer injury and mal-adaptive symptoms commonly referred to as over-training syndrome.

For everyone, the limiting factor in strength training is how frequently and intensely one can train without hurting one's progress…too often or too intensely risks injury and illness.

Consuming the B.N.B.B.s makes it possible to train at higher levels, more intensely, more frequently and with greater duration resulting in faster, more consistent gains in strength, with less likelihood of injury than people whom withhold the B.N.B.B.s, from their body.

Reason 24. To gain lean mass:

Gaining lean mass is similar to getting stronger, in that without a surplus of B.N.B.B.s in the body adequate and appropriate exercise, the lean tissue (all healthy tissue including bone, muscle, organs, immune system, reproductive system, nervous system, cardiovascular system, skin, sensory system, digestive system, respiratory system, hormone system and so on), simply won't improve to their full potential.

In fact, without adequate 1) Whole-foods 2) Functional-foods *and* 3) B.N.B.B.s (the three-parts of a complete nutrition program), exercise simply increases stress in the body and in simple terms, uses the body up from the inside out, promoting catabolism (breaking down of the body).

Most people think that exercising is good for the body and to a point it is. *BUT,* without Whole-foods, Functional-foods and B.N.B.B.s, exercise equates to driving your automobile, without putting adequate fuel in the tank and oil in the engine.

When we go on a trip we don't put the minimum amount of fuel in the tank just to get by, we fill the tank because there may be factors on the road which we can't plan for, that may use more fuel than the actual miles, from point-A-to-point-B.

Building lean mass is similar, in that there really are too many factors that go on in the body, at all different times, during any given 24-hour period, so it just makes sense to have the nutritional gas tank topped off, *at all times.*

The people whom emphasize exercise and play-with-fire, by skipping or skimping on the B.N.B.B.s, often are not only *dis-satisfied* with their lack of progress, but tend to complain of premature aging, knaggy injuries and lack of 'pep' as well as develop new back injuries, lose motivation and feel perplexed, as to why they are not only lacking progress, but even losing lean mass as they go along...*exercise does not equate to gaining lean mass!*

Building lean mass is the result of adequate, but not too much exercise, supported by adequate nutritional-resources on board, before the exercise (pre-workout), during and immediately afterward (post-workout), and in preparation for the next event and/or training session(s). The most lean and healthy people know this and apply these nutritional phenomena and earn seemingly extraordinary results. The people whom consider sensible-supplementation as "extreme" are the same people whom can't control cravings, *"...can never eat just one,"* and constantly complaining they, *"...aren't getting the results they should, for the amount of time, and energy they are putting into their workouts".* Without adequate nutrition (Whole-foods, Functional-foods and B.N.B.B.s), exercise without nutrition-density equates to 'going-through-the-motions'.

Reason 25. For more energy:

Once the body has utilized the B.N.B.B.s to make corrections (first in the DNA and the chemistry of the body), the body continues on making corrections and repairs in the body at the cellular-level...*nature decides on the priorities* and what areas of the body needs the nutrition-density...then, as corrections and repairs are made, it moves on to the next priority, *designated by nature.* **This is assuming you are consistent, in putting the nutrition in your body!**

The net result of good health, especially with a good, healthy surplus of , is more energy…not a jittery, caffeine/sugar, hyped-up type of energy that falls off and leaves you feeling emotionally down, but a healthy kind of energy that doesn't fluctuate from hour-to-hour. A consistent, predictable flow of energy that routinely provides an extra four-hours of energy, in the afternoon, when under-nourished folks hit-a-lull.

Remember!…the body has to use the nutrition to get itself healthy, at the cell level first, before you'll feel an improvement in energy…*energy comes from the cells and if they aren't healthy you won't have more energy until they are!* **Be consistent.**

Reason 26. To reduce pain & inflammation:

When the body is deficient of the B.N.B.B.s it will often be prone to inflammation and pain. That's just the way it is…*primed for inflammation.* A benefit of getting the B.N.B.B.s, in your body every day, is that *they subdue the inflammation process.* In other words, a side effect of not having enough B.N.B.B.s is inflammation, whether in the form of a *dis*-ease like arthritis or irritable bowel or in the case of inflammation that doesn't subside following trauma or injury the way it's supposed to. The person whom doesn't eat the B.N.B.B.s every day is primed for inflammation…***put them in your body and let nature take over.***

Reason 27. For more rapid healing:

Ok folks, *think about it*…your body is made of the B.N.B.B.s and if you don't put them in your body, so nature can utilize them to do routine repair, where in the heck is the body going to get them when healing needs the raw-materials, to permit healing to occur?

When nature is working to health the body it taps into the nutritional-resources on board, to rebuild the body. If they aren't there to tap into, ahead of time, the body has to delay healing to the rate at which you put them in, with whatever food stuff you consume. The higher the quality, the more nutrient-dense the product, the more accessible the nutrition is to the body. *If you care about your body, I recommend having them on board for whatever may arise.*

Reason 28. For faster recovery from exercise:

If you want to get the most fast and complete results from your exercise sessions, I suggest you make it a conscious, daily habit to put the B.N.B.B.s in your body, every day. If you don't it will take about four-times as long to get the same level of results, from your exercise and training, as someone whom is getting the B.N.B.B.s throughout each day (*especially with fat-loss efforts*).

That being said, that means what one person will accomplish in one-month will take the person nutritionally short four-months (that's neither a joke nor an exaggeration) and whatever the nutrient-deficient person does attain won't be sustainable, without them.

When we exercise, there is a period of time that the body repairs and makes stronger the areas of the body, which were stressed, by the exercise. *That's the adaptation process.* The body uses the nutrition, that is in the body ahead of time, to make stronger the body following exercise, but the body redirects the nutrition it would have used to maintain and repair the body to the more immediate need of repair and recovery of body systems, following exercise.

In short, without the sensible, supplemental B.N.B.B.s on board, nature has to decide between complete repair and maintenance of the body systems, repair of exercised body parts or partial repair of all the other systems of the body.

What typically happens with folks whom don't supplement their nutrition is that they start out looking good and strong, but as the days and weeks go by, their recovery wanes, their motivation drops off and they begin showing signs of over-training (such as knee problems, catching a cold bug and back pain), even though they are doing minimum workouts…they don't have enough nutrition on board! Then they have trouble maintaining the intensity and frequency of the workouts they built up to, within the first few months and complain of the knee hurting, then the elbow, then the low back and so on. I try to explain the connection between pain and random injuries, but to the people whom think sensible-supplementation is too much trouble or extreme, the pain and injuries will be a mystery! *Think about it.*

How that shows up in real time, is their strength drops off, they start catching colds that linger, they don't feel as great either before or after exercise. Especially the people whom say they don't believe in (or resist the idea of) nutritional supplements! They'll insist they aren't getting the kind of results they used to, but often continue to withhold Whole-foods, Functional-foods and the B.N.B.B.s.

The scientific definition of muscle recovery is the replenishment of protein and carbohydrates after exercise. So, what about all the other nutrients the rest of the body needs, outside of exercise?

Once people get the B.N.B.B.s in their body, on a consistent basis, it's like the lights have just been turned back on. From their complexion and attitude to their body fat and lean mass levels, to the blood chemistry levels all continue to improve…they can't believe it!…*"Sov, you won't believe what happened!"*

Reason 29. For greater mental capacity:

The brain…the most important organ of the body for health and vitality uses about 25% of the energy of the body…**yet, unlike every other system of the body, it doesn't store substantial energy for its own use!** The brain has to use what nutrition-density that happens to be circulating in the blood stream throughout the day. *Think about it…if it isn't circulating then the brain doesn't get any!*

How does the nutrition-density get into your bloodstream?

You have to put the nutrition-density, into your body everyday: 1) Whole-foods 2) Functional-foods and 3) The B.N.B.B.s. These are the only ways nutrition gets into the body…*you put it in your body and let nature take over.*

In other words, the better nutrition has been stored up in the cells of the body, the more will be available for the brain.

A person that hears and sees what would help them and even has a person whom is willing to coach and morally support them in the process, yet still doesn't take action has more problems than I can help them with…because they have something big that they have to work out for themselves…*like a chip on the shoulder.* So, do it. You'll have a lot more mental energy and capacity…or don't, *it's up to you.*

Daniel Amen, MD, psychiatrist, PBS feature speaker and author of *Change Your Mind, Change You Life* says, "…*nutrition is a major factor in the health of the structure AND the ability of the brain to function optimally is dependant on nutritional supplements."* (The B.N.B.B.s).

Amen says, *"When you optimize your brain, everything in your life is better."*

Reason 30. Significant improvement in endurance:

Just like strength, lean mass, bone mass, weight-loss and energy improvement, endurance is all the net result of having good health, as a result of surplus nutritional-resources. If you only have the minimum in your gas tank, you'll never have near the endurance you *could* have.

People whom have been training consistently and eating fairly clean leading up to adding Functional-foods and B.N.B.B.s, generally have personal best performances, *within the first week.*

Reason 31. Peace of mind:

In my extensive experience, I have realized that the two most significant factors for health assurance are 1) how the individual operates their mind, *e.g. Do they practice optimism and 2) what do they put in their body nutritionally?* Do they put the B.N.B.B.s in?

When you put the B.N.B.B.s in your body every day, other than an optimistic, looking-forward-to-a-bright-future, the glass-is-refillable attitude, you can have peace of mind that you are taking care of the two most important factors which contribute to long-term good health...*your mind and your lifestyle.*

Reason 32. Eat less than 10-servings of fruit each day?

That's part of what it takes to get enough nutrition every day. Skip a day? You're off track. Make up the difference by putting the B.N.B.B.s in your body and ***let nature take over.***

Reason 33. Eat less than 10-servings of vegetables each day?

That's part of what it takes to get enough nutrition every day. Skip a day? You're off track. Make up the difference with the convenience of the B.N.B.B.s. Put them in and **let nature take over**...*it's that easy.*

Reason 34. Have been taking poor quality, synthetic or extracted supplements, until now?

As you know from my previous books and lectures and whether your ego is interfering with your ability to process truth or not, poor-quality dietary-supplements don't provide nutritional support to the cells adequately for them to reproduce healthy versions of themselves. There is a portion of the population whom really doesn't care if they get nutrition-density or not and this shows up by consuming poor-quality supplement, just so they can *say they are taking something.* For those kinds of personalities there's not much I can do for them, since they have a different value system; *they make purchases based on what is cheap or advertised the most or what their insurance will cover versus a value of aiming to put the highest quality nutrition into the body.* I specialize in coaching/training people whom value quality over cheapness. It's very easy for me, after decades of this, to make recommendations that I guarantee your satisfaction and that is one thing I offer my clients.

The difference that makes the difference:

A study I read once talked about experiments on the ocean's water ability to support life. Some scientists took a sample of ocean water and tested it attempting to identify all the ingredients (the ones that had been identified). Then they took fresh water and added in all those ingredients they were able to identify which they found in the ocean water. Then they placed some creatures that lived in the ocean water in the 'man-made' water. All the creatures died. The experiment was repeated a number of times, with the same results.

Eventually, the scientists began adding the actual ocean water into the fresh water to find out how much would be needed to again, support life. To their dismay, only a fraction of ocean water was needed, to support life [and the 'ingredients' which were missing in the fresh water were not identifiable, nor duplicable, with the testing equipment that was developed at that time]. You see the ocean's ability to create life is beyond what modern science has learned to measure with its equipment and machines. Nutrition is similar in this way. *Supplemental B.N.B.B.s that only contain the known factors (vitamins, minerals, etc.), do not produce near the results of B.N.B.B.s that are processed in such a way to preserve the unknown factors.*

Examples from other mammals:

Although I don't condone animal testing, I find the following example rather relevant: Dr. Pottinger did a 10-year study on 900 cats, back in the 1940's.

First, he fed the cats a diet of raw food. The cats reproduced normally, with an average litter of five, for each generation. The babies nursed normally, had excellent equilibrium and predictable behavior.

Then he fed the cats cooked food. As a result, each kitten had different and abnormal skeletal development. The spontaneous abortion rate was 25% with the first generation of kittens. Meaning 25% of the first set spontaneously aborted their babies, before full-term. By just the second-generation, the spontaneous abortion rate was 70%. Often the babies died of malnutrition because they were too weak to nurse and often the mother died within three-months of giving birth, being fed the cooked food.

The female cats were irritable and dangerous to handle.

The males became docile and their sex drive dropped off. Parasitic infestation increased in the cats fed cooked food. Skin problems and allergies were frequent and progressively worse with each generation.

By the third-generation, none of the cats lived to the sixth-month.

It took four-generations, of the cats being fed raw food, before they regenerated significantly.

Lifecycle of cats:

Another study went something like this:

A family of cats had just one-or-two essential nutrients withheld, from their diet, every day.

The 1st-generation had less shine to their fur.

The 2nd-generation had less shine to their fur *and they required more sleep.*

The 3rd-generation had less shine to their fur, *slept more and lost their sight earlier in life.*

The 4th-generation had less shine to their fur, *slept more, lost their sight earlier and developed immune system problems.*

The 5th-generation had less shine to their fur, *slept more, lost their sight earlier, developed immune system problems and couldn't reproduce.*

Is this making sense?

Top 10 Dietary-supplements as described on WebMD:

Whether they really need them or not, sales figures show that plenty of people are purchasing supplements. Here are some of the most popular supplement categories:

Multi-vitamins:

Taking a daily Multi-vitamin with minerals has long been considered nutritional 'insurance' to cover dietary shortfalls.

"There is no harm in taking a once-daily multivitamin, as long as you select one based on your age and sex," says Grotto. *"Take one daily or just on days when your diet is inadequate."*

Meal replacements (Functional-foods):

Powdered and liquid products...might not be what most of us think of as dietary-supplements. But they're included in the list because they are designed to supplement the diet (diet is also known as Whole-foods). For people whom can't eat regular food because of illnesses, these products are good alternatives. And what about weight management? Using a meal replacement can help control calories and be beneficial, experts say -- as long as it's part of a lifestyle that includes exercise.

Sports nutrition supplements (Functional-foods):

This is a broad category that includes both sports performance and weight-loss supplements. It includes pills, powders, formulas and drinks formulated not just to hydrate but to enhance physical activity. Among them are protein formulas.

"These products provide a subtle, incremental effect. You can't use a sports supplement for a week and expect to gain pounds of muscle, but if used properly, research shows they can provide a slight, not overwhelming, edge," says Andrew Shoa, PhD, vice president for regulatory affairs for the Council for Responsible Nutrition, a trade association for the dietary-supplement industry.

In my experience, **the kind I use can provide a 20%-50% improvement, in fitness, performance, fat-loss and overall well-being.**

Kris Clark, PhD, RD, Sports Nutrition Director at Penn State University, says she very carefully uses select sports supplements with collegiate athletes: *"I rely on the major nutrients in food, timing of meals and fluids to enhance athletic performance, and in general ...after practice or events for muscle cell recovery."*

Calcium:

Calcium is one of the minerals most often lacking in Americans' diets.

B-Complex:

B-Complex vitamins include Biotin, Thiamin, Niacin, Riboflavin, Pantothenic Acid, Vitamin B-6, Choline, Inositol and Vitamin B-12.

Some people say, *"Many of us don't need these supplements,"* which is a common mantra, but when you look at all the groups that do need supplements, its more people than those whom do not need supplements (B.N.B.B.s).

"One exception," **he says,** *"...is seniors, whom may need additional B-12 because as we get older, we absorb less of it. People with certain medical conditions or whom take drugs that interfere with vitamin absorption may also require supplementation (yet, three more groups whom need supplements!)."*

Vitamin C:

Vitamin C is often taken in an effort to ward off colds.

"...it won't do any harm..," Grotto says, *"Because it is a water-soluble vitamin, (it isn't stored in the body) and excess amounts are simply excreted. Your health-care provider may tell*

you to take Vitamin C if you have a wound that's healing," (**oh look! yet,** *another* **group whom needs supplemental B.N.B.B.s).**

Glucosamine and Chondroitin:

These supplements are often taken by people with joint pain.

Results in a subgroup of study participants, with moderate to severe pain showed the combination may be effective. While the evidence is not conclusive enough to some experts, some rheumatologists say many of their patients find relief from the com bination. *"About 40% of my osteoarthritis patients benefit from taking 1,500 mg of glucosamine and 1,200 mg chondroitin sulphate a day (for) 4-to-8 weeks,"* says Kaiser Permanente rheumatologist Eduardo Baetti, MD.

Vitamin D:

Chances are, you are not getting enough Vitamin D for good health.

"The current recommendations are not adequate to protect against chronic dis-eases or prevent osteoporosis," Vitamin D expert Michael Holick, MD, tells WebMD. Holick suggests taking a daily Vitamin D supplement.

Fish/animal oil:

"95% of the sales in this category come from fish and not animal oils," says Rea Clark will continue to recommend fatty-acids supplements because *"...most people don't come near meeting the American Heart Association recommendations, for fatty-fish twice-weekly, and with a heightened fear of mercury levels in all types of fish, people are not coming close to getting enough Omega-3 in their diets."*

As a side note, the kind of fish and plant oils I personally use are free of mercury and other toxins and I'm happy to share them with you as a client of mine. My contact information is in the appendix.

Chapter Five

Animals are different?

With cats and other domesticated animals, like dogs, horses and cows, which have a much shorter lifespan, we get to witness the complete cycle of effects, of inadequate-nutrition, relatively quickly, from birth-to-death. From one-generation-to-the-next, the effects show up very quickly. Because we live longer than those animals, we have the opportunity to witness the lifespan effects of inadequate nutrition, from-beginning-to-end. We get to see the effects for ourselves, the effects of eating substandard food, over a lifetime, in only a fraction of our own lifetime. Cats can reproduce five-generations, in a-year-or-two and their entire life may exist over 20-years.

J.I. Rodale, The American Naturalist, wrote in his book *The Complete Book of Food and Nutrition*:

"We must take vitamins if we wish to be healthy and the nation as a whole must do it, or God alone knows what will happen to the second or third-generation coming up...generations inheriting weaknesses passed on to them by us, generations which few of us will live to see, unless we augment our diet with vitamins and minerals."

Reason 35. Gaps between what we should be eating and what we actually eat:

We know we should be eating good, but we don't always eat what we should. B.N.B.B.s make up the nutritional difference [at a fraction of the cost] of equivalent amounts of Whole-foods and more conveniently...***just put them in and let nature do the rest.***

Reason 36. Have been eating by hypothetical-nutrition standards/theory-based nutrition:

The standards set by the government to meet our daily nutritional requirements are too low for optimizing health, breaking the cycle of chronic *dis*-ease, fat-loss and athletic performance.

During 1977 and 1978 a document called *The Anarem Report* was published in conjunction with the United States Department of Agriculture. 21,500 people were surveyed* about what they ate during a three-day period. The report revealed that not a single person got 100% of even the minimums of Vitamins A, B6, B12, Thiamin, Riboflavin, Vitamin-C, minerals Calcium, Magnesium, Iron nor Protein (not even in relation to those 1930's and 1940's food data bases that are supposed to know what we are eating). All of these nutrients are essential to the body and are some of what I consider the B.N.B.B.s and to get the benefits I offer you in this book (some of the so-called experts would consider this information inaccurate because they survey people asking them to recall what they ate in the previous three-days, stating people can't remember that far back).

*A similar survey was performed 10-years later and the results were not much better. 70% of men and 80% of women did not get even 2/3 of the daily minimums.

I will not say that *no one gets what they need from food*, I simply do not know anyone whom does...do you?...How would we know?

Whom else isn't getting enough nutrition, based on government standards?

According to Dr. Ruth Weir of the Department of Agriculture, not one group (children, teens, adults or seniors), was getting their minimum requirements, on a daily basis.

A newspaper article I read in a Tacoma, Washington newspaper reported that 60% of children entering kindergarten were nutritionally anemic, deficient in one-or-more of the nutrients tested for.

The Center for Disease Control (CDC) reported 700,000 children aged one-to-two-years old are nutritionally anemic.

According to the United States Department of Agriculture, 75% of children eat less than one vegetable *per day*. Most whom are considered to eat vegetables are counting potato chips, french-fries and ketchup as vegetables.

The CDC reported nearly 8-million teenage women are nutritionally-anemic. Another study showed that 68% were deficient in at least *some* of the essential nutrients at levels designed as 'minimum', ***if it were in the food to begin with.***

The Third Report on Nutritional Monitoring in the United States Executive Summary 1995, commissioned by the United States Department of Agriculture and Department of Health and Human Services, showed that less than 30% of American adults meet the 'minimum' recommendations for fruit and vegetable consumption, missing out on the chemical protective effect (cancer prevention effects).

A Tacoma, Washington Newspaper reported in June 1999 an Associated Press article entitled, *"Delivered meals fail to stop senior's malnourishment."*

Marcia Stein, President of the New York Meals on Wheels said, *"Malnourishment among the elderly is a serious national epidemic."*

Denise Martin, Director of Development for Rhode Island Meals on Wheels said, *"It's [malnourishment] a major crisis...we serve 900 people each week and we have over 300 on the waiting list whom are ill and the problem is getting worse."*

Vivien keys, Director of Wake County, North Carolina Meals on Wheels estimated, *"...52% of its recipients are at risk for malnourishment...most are over 80-years old and only the most at risk get two-meal- a-day and 41% of U.S. cities have waiting lists."*

In 1996 the Associated Press reported on the escalation and fueling of city violence, crime rates, health costs, poor school work and obesity [as a result of inadequate nutrition].

Research from the UK suggests that consistent consumption of nutritional supplements can reduce violent behavior; Investigators tested the effects of vitamins and mineral supplements, as well as essential fatty-acids (good fats), from fish, on 231 men – all maximum-security prisoners. 1/2 the men took daily nutritional supplements, and the other half took a placebo. Even after two-weeks of supplement use, the University of Surrey in Guilford, England reported that prisoners whom were given a range of vitamins and nutrients, commonly found in produce, with their food showed a [37% reduction in antisocial behavior including violence].

Dr. Stephan Davies of London's Biolab Medical Unit analyzed 65,000 samples of blood, hair and sweat over a 15-year period. Without exception, when results were compared with the ages of patients the levels of the toxic, anti-nutrients lead, cadmium, aluminum and mercury had increased *while the levels of the health-building minerals such as Magnesium, Zinc, Chromium and Selenium had decreased.*

The Public Health Institute, The California Department of Health Services, The California Children's Eating and Exercise Survey in conjunction with The California Division of The American Cancer Society found in their study that four-out-of-five children, in the 9-to-11 age group did not eat fruits and vegetables every day, *missing out on the nutritional basics on a regular basis.*

In 1985 *The Bateman Report* found that more than 85% of people whom generally thought they ate a well-balanced diet failed to meet the recommended daily allowance levels. *That is 85% of people do not even get the minimum amounts, of the B.N.B.B.s.*

In 1988 the *Surgeon General Report on Nutrition and Health Summary and Records from the U.S. Department of Health and*

Human Services reported, *"... diet influences disease and health in a major way...of the 2.2 million whom die each year, 1.8 million are diet-related...eradicate these and you instantly extend your probable healthy lifespan by 10-to-25 years...by preventing these diseases and all the degenerative changes that lead up to them, you effectively turn back the clock and slow down the aging process."*

Sooo, it sounds like there's some more groups that don't get enough from food!

Reason 37. Are taking prescription medications?

All prescription medications have side-effects, *that's a known fact.* One of the side-effects is that certain medications deplete certain B.N.B.B.s from the body, raising the level of the B.N.B.B.s needed by the body.

The Nutritional Cost of Drugs: A Guide to Maintaining Good Nutrition While Using Prescription and Over-The-Counter Drugs and *The Drug-Nutrient Depletion Guide* are just two-books, which demonstrate which B.N.B.B.s get depleted, by each category of prescription drugs. There are numerous works that have shown that each drug depletes *some* of the minimum nutrition we get, from the food we eat...assuming we have enough nutrition-density, in our body to begin with,...or that it's in the soil and food to begin with...*get that loop?*

Many of the most common *de*-generative *dis*-eases we recognize today are largely based on lack of nutrition-density in the daily dietary habits and lack of exercise...so, taking drugs to cover up the symptoms of lack of nutrition and then those very drugs deplete nutrition-density even more...*does that make any sense at all?*

Now here's a very important point I want you to get: If you are on prescription-medication you're not necessarily a healthy person. The more medications you are taking, the unhealthier you may be. You're taking the medications because you have some *dis*-ease occurring in your body as it is, *which means your requirements for the B.N.B.B.s may be higher than a healthy person,* right from the get-go. Medications which deplete nutrients from the body increase the need for the B.N.B.B.s, even more...government minimum requirements don't even come close.

Prescription medications, for the most part, are a great way to control the symptoms until the lifestyle factors that created the health problem to begin with are improved...that's your job, not your doctor's job.

I'm not saying stop taking your medications cold-turkey...that could likely be a dangerous proposition. The medications control the symptoms of poor, sub-par lifestyle habits. Ideally, you'll want to talk to your physician(s), tell them you want their support in reducing medications that might be dangerous and you would like their help monitoring your health while you improve your daily lifestyle habits (improve your nutritional and exercise habits). If your physician can't help you, you may want to get a second-opinion or a third-opinion, from a professional whom has helped others do the same thing...they are out there, so shop around until you find the one who knows what you need to know.

B.N.B.B.s are not a treatment for *dis*-ease or *de*-generative problems. When a person doesn't have enough B.N.B.B.s the body begins to slowly or quickly break down from-the-inside-out and the signs and symptoms show up as *dis*-eases like heart *dis*-ease, obesity, high blood pressure, high cholesterol, fatigue, mental fogginess, depression and the like. Conventional medical care's strength is emergency medicine, keeping people alive when trauma and emergency strike. But there's nothing more a doctor can do if you aren't taking care of yourself on a daily basis...*your lifestyle*. That means not eating junk food, eating more Whole-foods & Functional-foods and sensible-supplementation of the B.N.B.B.s to make up for gaps in what some would consider a balanced diet.

As an individual, you'll have to decide whether it makes sense to you or not that the food alone you are eating is enough to support the cells of your body. Do you have the health you want?

If health professionals tell you that they, *"...don't believe in supplements,"* ask them if they are taking the B.N.B.B.s. If they aren't then they aren't really talking about their personal-experience, they are talking about what they wish was true or what *they think* is the responsible thing to tell you, without really knowing any better.

Every physician, pharmacist and nurse knows that drugs have side-effects, but not every nurse or physician has personally experienced the benefits of the B.N.B.B.s.

Doctors are often skeptical about the B.N.B.B.s and I don't blame them one bit. I do know physicians whom put the B.N.B.B.s in their own body (having personal-experience with them) and consider them preventive maintenance versus medical treatment. Surprising to me is how common it is for neurologists and psychiatrists to put the B.N.B.B.s in their body and recommend them to their patients. I think part of the reason is that they routinely see the brain scans of people whom think they get enough from food and the differences in the patients' brains in the ones whom do put the B.N.B.B.s in their body, allowing the nutrition-density to circulate, through the brain. The differences show up on brain scans! Dr. Amen on PBS shows examples of brains with and without adequate nutrition on his television specials. Brain scans of individuals whom are addicts also show a 'shrinking' of the important gray matter of the front of the brain, *as is common for under-nourished individuals.*

Medical treatment comes when you don't take care of your body's nutritional needs consistently enough that your body breaks down and you have to go get drugs to cover up the symptoms of the underlying deficiency. Doctors are amazingly intelligent and committed individuals, but there are so many dietary-supplement scams out there, nowadays, that until they use good ones they won't have any positive things to tell you about them nor encourage you to take them. Statistically, a thousand supplement companies start up and go out of business each year! There's on average 85,000 different supplements on the market at any given time, many of which are either extracted or synthetic. Supplement companies come and go, partly, due to poor business practices, but partly because demand exceeds the available supplies to make good B.N.B.B.s. The ones I take have been around for a what I would consider a very long time (60-years), and I've been successfully using them for 26-years.

Truth is that people whom haven't taken good care of themselves and their body is breaking down often don't even comply with the doctor's orders for prescription drugs, so it's not likely someone is going to take optional dietary-supplements if they won't even commit to take the medication that could save their life...you can't save everyone! If I were a doctor and had a patient whom wouldn't comply, I wouldn't likely recommend something that could take even longer to help the body if the patient wouldn't take the quick-fix prescription.

The April 1998 issue of *The American Medical Association* published an article about prescription drugs. There are, on average, over 2,000,000 adverse drug reactions [reported] each year requiring hospitalization, prolonged hospitalization and permanent *dis*-ability. On average 106,000 people die each year, in hospitals, from prescription drugs that are [properly prescribed]. Ten-years ago, properly prescribed medications were known to be the 4th leading cause of death in the U.S.

In 1987 – the only year it has done so – The Food and Drug Administration asked all physicians in Rhode Island to report all 'adverse events' from medications in the previous year. Surveyed directly, doctors reported 27,000 cases, as opposed to the 55-cases, listed that year, by the FDA's voluntary reporting system.

There are no deaths from eating the B.N.B.B.s, the way I recommend.

When the diabetes drug Rezulin was withdrawn in March 2000, the FDA announced that it had been linked to 63 confirmed deaths from liver damage, although the agency's own senior drug safety specialist calculated that more than 400 occurred.

Does it make sense to you to prevent *dis*-ease, rather than eating yourself into *dis*-ease and then taking drugs that are supposed to cover up the symptoms, only to die from the toxicity of the drug that even the doctors are not informed of?

An upcoming chapter is about possible reasons why your doctor hasn't talked with you about the B.N.B.B.s.

The clincher here is that all prescription drugs have side-effects. The B.N.B.B.s do not...*hmmm.*

Reason 38. Thought you could get all you needed from the food you eat?

If you have any health problems, its likely your body's requirements for nutrition are greater then you or your medical team know (greater than the minimum amounts the government recommends...think about it...every increase in nutrition-density the government might recommend decreases the profits for food and drug manufacturers...get it? Since there is no downside to the consumer taking the B.N.B.B.s there's no risk giving them a three, four or five-month test on yourself. Personally, I work with clients whom think long-term and are willing to commit for a year. Although you'll notice some of the benefits within a few days, it takes about a year to rebuild every part of the body and I don't want you to miss out on any of that.

Reason 39. Been living by the 'as if' diet?

The 'as-if' diet is when people think they are eating enough Whole-foods, based on what a data base or book speculates on how much nutrition is any given food item.

In reality, the only way to know how much nutrition is in the food you ate is to test the food before you eat it. The only assurance you are getting enough B.N.B.B.s is to supplement with the B.N.B.B.s in sensible ways.

Theo Clark, Ph.D., visiting chemistry professor at Truman State University found that organic oranges contain up to 30% more nutrition than conventional-farming. *"Because conventional oranges are larger than organic fruit and have a deeper color, we were expecting twice as much Vitamin C in the conventional oranges,"* Dr. Clark says.

On March 7, 2003, U.S. researchers reported that organically-grown crops contain more healthy compounds than conventional-crops. *"Tests on organically and sustainably grown corn and berries showed they contain 50%-to-58% more polyphenolics (the compounds that act as antioxidants and may protect cells against damage that can lead to the heart dis-ease and cancer) (the de-generative dis-eases so popular, in America today), than conventionally grown food,"* said Alyson Mitchell, an Assistant Professor of Food Science at the University of California, Davis, whom led the study.

WebMd posted an article written by Peter Jaret and Reviewed by Arefa Cassoobhoy, MD, MPH, entitled *Older Adults: 9-Nutrients You May Be Missing.*

(When reading this brief overview, see if you notice any similarities of opinions of which B.N.B.B.s might be consistent themes).

Even then, you may fall short. *"As we get older, the body becomes less efficient at absorbing some key nutrients,"* says Katherine Tucker, RD, PhD, chair of the department of health sciences at Northeastern University in Boston. *"In addition, the ability to taste food declines, blunting appetite. Some foods become difficult to chew or digest."*

Several key nutrients in particular may be in short supply as you get older. Here are the top vitamins and nutrients to look out for -- and how to get enough.

Vitamin B12 (one of the B-complex):

B12 is important for creating red blood cells and DNA, and for maintaining healthy nerve function. *"Getting enough B12 is a challenge for older people because they can't absorb it from food as well as younger people,"* says Tucker. *"Even if your diet contains enough, you may be falling short."*

Folate/Folic Acid (one of the B-complex):

You may have heard of Folate. Too little of this essential B Vitamin is known for contributing to anemia and increasing the risk of a pregnant woman having a baby with a neural tube defect. Older people whose diets don't include a lot of fruits and vegetables or fortified breakfast cereals may be falling short.

Calcium:

Calcium plays many roles in the body. But, it is most important for building and maintaining strong bones. Unfortunately, surveys show that as we age, we consume less Calcium in our diets. *"Calcium is so essential that if you don't get enough, your body will leach it out of your bones,"* says Zelman. Coming up short on Calcium has been shown to increase the risk of brittle bones and fractures.

Calcium continued...

How to hit the mark: *"The body needs both calcium and protein for bone health,"* says Heaney. *"If you tend to steer clear of dairy products, talk to your doctor about whether you should take a supplement."* (See that again? Referring to a doctor whom doesn't necessarily have any nutrition training...why is that?)

Joanne Koenig Coste, a former caregiver whom works with older people says, *"...smoothies made with yogurt, fruit, and even vegetables can be an attractive option for people whom have lost their appetite, have trouble chewing, or have a dry mouth. I used to make one for my mother with spinach, yogurt, a little orange juice, and a little pistachio ice cream,"* she says. *"My mother loved it. I'd divide it into small portions and freeze them for her. She'd take it out in the morning and have it for lunch."*

Personally, I use GMO free protein, yogurt and frozen fruit with some added water to make a fast, convenient smoothie I can drink throughout the day. If you want extra help with this, during your consultation, I'm happy to share my favorite recipes with you.

Vitamin D:

"Vitamin D helps the body absorb Calcium, maintain bone density, and prevent osteoporosis," says Zelman. Recent findings suggest that Vitamin D may also protect against some chronic *diseases*, including cancer, Type 1 diabetes, rheumatoid arthritis, multiple sclerosis, depression and autoimmune diseases. In older people, Vitamin D deficiency has also been linked to increased risk of falling. Many Americans fall short on Vitamin D, which is mainly produced by the skin when exposed to sunlight. Many experts think older people need to take Vitamin D supplements, since the skin becomes less efficient at producing the vitamin from sunlight as we age.

Potassium:

Getting enough Potassium in your diet may also help keep bones strong. This essential mineral is vital for cell function and has also been shown to help reduce high blood pressure and the risk of kidney stones. Unfortunately, surveys show that many older Americans don't get the recommended 4,700 mg of Potassium a day.

Magnesium:

Magnesium plays a crucial role in some 300 different physiological processes. Getting enough can help keep your immune system in top shape, your heart healthy, and your bones strong. *"Many Whole-foods, including vegetables, contain magnesium. [But it is often lost in processing],"* says Tucker. Absorption of Magnesium decreases with age. Some medications older people take, including diuretics, may also reduce Magnesium absorption.

Fiber:

Fiber helps promote healthy digestion by moving foods through the digestive tract. Foods rich in fiber, including whole-grains, beans, fruits, and vegetables, have many other health benefits, including protecting against heart *dis*-ease. *"If you don't eat a lot of these Whole-foods, chances are you're not getting enough fiber,"* says Zelman. *"You're not alone. [Most Americans only get about half the recommended levels]."*

Omega-3 Fats:

These unsaturated fats, found primarily in fish, have a wide range of benefits, including possibly reducing symptoms in rheumatoid arthritis and slowing the progression of age-related macular degeneration, a *dis*-ease of reduced vision in the elderly. *"New evidence suggests that Omega-3s may also reduce the risk of Alzheimer's dis-ease and perhaps even keep the brain sharper as we age,"* says Zelman. Seafood should be part of a heart-healthy diet.

How to hit the mark: Nutrition experts recommend helping yourself to at least two servings of fish a week. Omega 3 supplements are available.

Water:

Water might not seem like an essential vitamin or mineral, but it is crucial for good health. With age, sense of thirst may decline. Certain medicines increase the risk for becoming dehydrated. Water is especially important if you are increasing the fiber in your diet, since it absorbs water. In the *Modified MyPyramid for Older Adults,* created by Tufts University Researchers, suggest 8-glasses of fluids, a day, are next to physical activity in importance for health, as well as dietary-supplements to make up for gaps in the diet, absorption problems and medications which can interfere with nutrient absorption.

Chapter Six

Do-over

Want to halt the *de*-generative *dis*-ease process? If you are already having some health problems, you may likely benefit from the B.N.B.B.s.

The process goes something like this:

When you start putting the B.N.B.B.s in your body and keep doing it consistently, the sequence of the process goes like this…

a) **Halt** the *dis*-ease or *de*-generation, of the body systems and capabilities,

b) **Prevent further damage,** from previous inadequate consumption, of the B.N.B.B.s,

c) **Begin reversing prior damage,** from inadequate B.N.B.B.s. and

d) **Repair, rebuild and maintain** the fundamental systems and capabilities of the body…*the point where personal performance will significantly improve beyond what you thought you were capable of.*

Want to reverse the *de*-generative *dis*-ease process? If you are already having some health problems, you may likely benefit from the B.N.B.B.s.

Reason 40. Have been chasing symptoms through the "Black-Forest" with 'medicinal' nutrition or prescription drugs?

You will often hear me refer to this as the "Black-Forest" of chasing symptoms. Often, in fairy-tales and sci-fi stories, they talk about places like the "Black- Forest". The only way to get through the "Black-Forest" is to stay on the path, no matter what you see or think you see or hear. If you get off the path, anything short of a miracle and you're lost forever. This same phenomenon occurs all the time in the medical-maze of chronic *dis*-ease. In fact, it is the basis of much medical treatment.

The right path being making sure you get enough B.N.B.B.s, regardless of what else is going on in life. *Simply put them in and let nature do the rest.*

Symptoms of illness or *dis*-ease can be considered the early warning signs of a problem. Much medical 'treatment' is putting chemicals into the body to cover up the very early warning-signs the body is giving to let us know there is a problem (great for trauma, emergencies, bleeding and fractures).

Once a drug is given to cover up the underlying symptom(s) the body has to find a different way to let you know of the problem. In addition, I know of no exception that every drug has side-effects, which in turn have to be covered up with more drugs. I have known of people on as many as 30-different prescriptions, all at the same time! My mom recently passed and was on 25-different prescriptions, at that time.

That is one-way people end up on so many different drugs and their health just keeps getting worse and worse. Some professionals try to utilize nutrition, as if it is chemical drugs. Nutrition doesn't work that way, but professionals often use this as rationale for presumed inconsistent results...meaning, they try to 'treat' health problems with nutrition, attempting to chase symptoms.

In the burning-house scenario, it would be like throwing lumber and other building materials on a hot fire. In the prescription drug scenario, it would be like filling the burning house with fire-retardant asbestos. Yes, the fire is out but now, the house is too toxic to inhabit. The patient ends up way off course, deep in the "Black-Forest" of chasing symptoms. *"Oh! There's one...there's another... and another!"*

Pretty soon, they find themselves hanging out with other people on the same drugs, comparing notes about which side-effects they are experiencing and being told they just have to learn to live with it as it is a *"...natural part of the aging process."*

Once a person ventures off the path of health and gets lost in the "Black-Forest" it can be very difficult to escape. Around every turn is another caring health professional telling you to just do what your doctor says. And they are so very convincing because they do really care about you and because as far as they know they are providing the highest quality information and care. And that is the clincher...*based on their experience,* they are giving you the very best information based on 'treating' symptoms. If I were severely injured in a car accident or any other type of emergency I would want to be right there in the emergency room with the highly trained experts in their field utilizing the most up to date and high-tech drugs and diagnostics to keep my heart pumping blood, until my body gets stabilized.

Emergencies, acute trauma, some surgery, illness and diagnostics are a few of the strengths of current medicine. Subacute and chronic *dis*-eases are offered little in the way of medicine and yes there are exceptions to this.

Reason 41. Prevent *dis*-ease:

Because parts of the medical establishment, whom are in the business to 'treat' *dis*-ease are not taught about the early warning signs of sub-clinical *mal*-nutrition and really, information to prevent sub-clinical *mal*-nutrition is sparse, to say the least, in this country. In some ways, doctors are kept separate from the information that would educate and empower them to notice which signs, symptoms, complaints, and *de*-generative *dis*-eases are rooted in basic lack of nutrition and exercise...the very information that would help doctors themselves!

One effect is that most of us are not taught to notice the slow, gradual effects and so it seems like health problems just happen *"...all of a sudden, out of nowhere"*. The truth is that most of the *de*-generative *dis*-eases occur in a step-by-step fashion, within the body...they are a controllable process that each person has a responsibility to. Heart *dis*-ease for example, preventable in some cases, is a 10-to-30-year process, of putting things in the body which stop blood flow to the heart, interrupt with proper functioning and capability of the circulatory system, while simultaneously withholding the B.N.B.B.s. Did you get that?

Reason 42. Catch small problems before they become big problems:

When the body does begin to break down, little knaggy problems pop up and they're commonly referred to as the, *"Normal aging process." Yes, they are normal... for people whom are not optimally nourished, every day!* Unfortunately, the usual standard for good health is based on people whom are getting just enough nutrition to be alive and free of major suffering, with the help of chemicals known as prescription drugs, to cover up the symptoms of subpar-nutrition we should be paying attention to.

The Washington Post article, By Jennifer LaRue Huget, published August 23, 2011, entitled *Dietary-supplements: Do we need them, or can we get all our nutrients from food?*

"In an ideal world, no one would need dietary-supplements. Our balanced diets would provide all the vitamins, minerals and other nutrients our bodies need...the latest federal data show that more than 1/2 of U.S. adults use dietary-supplements, mostly Multi-vitamins."

"A fundamental premise of the Dietary Guidelines is that nutrients should come primarily from foods. But, as I wrote in 2009, meeting your daily dietary needs, without using supplements is a challenge, even when you're choosing ultra-healthful foods, under a professional dietitian's guidance. It's a widespread challenge. Society has "...invested a lot in the science behind the Dietary Guidelines for Americans,"" says Duffy MacKay, vice president for scientific and regulatory affairs for the Council for Responsible Nutrition.

"When you think about people and what they're eating, a significant number are not meeting those benchmarks," says MacKay.

Robert Post, Deputy Director of the U.S. Department of Agriculture's Center for Nutrition Policy and Promotion, says,

"...too few Americans are meeting all their nutritional requirements and that dietary-supplements, used sensibly, can help fill gaps in our diets." In particular, he notes, the guidelines single out, *"...four nutrients of concern,"* that most of us need more of to maintain good health: Potassium, Vitamin D, Calcium and Fiber.

Roberta Anding, Director of Sports Nutrition at Texas Children's Hospital and a spokeswoman for the American Dietetic Association, advises consulting an expert to determine the types and quantities of supplements that might benefit you.

MacKay, whose job might seem to require him to push supplements over food, observes that good nutrition is, *"...not an either-or-situation."*

"Focus on food, first. Maintain a varied diet," (Whole-foods), MacKay suggests. *"Once you take a snapshot of your diet, then figure out where to supplement to make sure you get everything you need."* (Functional-foods and B.N.B.B.s).

The USDA is adamant that people try to get the Fiber, Potassium, Vitamin D and Calcium they need by eating more fruits and vegetables. But the Harvard School of Public Health suggests a daily Multi-vitamin, calling it, *"...a great nutrition insurance policy."*

MacKay agrees with that approach. *"A Multi-vitamin can smooth the 'ups and downs of diet',"* he says. *"It's not a magic bullet, and it's not promising anything, just filling in."*

Retrieved from:
https://www.washingtonpost.com/lifestyle/wellness/dietary-supplements-do-we-need-them-or-can-we-get-all-our-nutrients-from-food/2011/08/18/gIQAAKlkYJ_story.html?utm_term=.ded432ab2042

This is why I approach it from this angle: A complete nutrition program includes three parts:

1) Whole-foods

2) Functional-foods and

3) B.N.B.B.s.

Whole-foods have to be the basis and foundation of good health. Functional-foods elicit certain responses, for example during fat-loss and athletics, where food alone doesn't work fast enough to do any good for fast, efficient and complete recovery from exercise & training (with weight-loss and athletics & fitness, timing is critical for maximum effectiveness), as well as keeping blood sugar/insulin levels stable to (maximize the fat-burning effects of resistance-training and fat-burning cardio), as well as "re-sensitizing" the body to insulin, (which is the essence of fast, safe and long-term, sustainable fat-loss), thereby eliminating insulin resistance, which is how Type-2 diabetes occurs in the body. And the B.N.B.B.s are to fill in gaps and make up for things that either increase one's need for nutrition and/or or to simply fill in the gaps from inconsistent eating habits.

Chapter Seven

What the heck happened?

Reason 43. Food changes in the last 100-years:

Here is what I found. Up until about the late 1800's much of the food in America was produced by farmers in rural communities. That means it was grown in smaller amounts and it was fresher because it was picked when ripe and sold locally. And there was very little processing done to the food, so it had all the nutrition-density retained/left in. But between the 1870's and early 1900's major food companies started buying and growing massive quantities of grains like wheat and processing them through their mills, in order to offer convenience and increase their profit. Basically, they began running the raw grains, the mainstay of much of what is called food today, through huge rollers or mills to process and remove the outer shell of the grain.

By removing the outer shell, or fiber, of the grain insects and rodents are less likely to eat it and makes for a longer shelf life and much higher profit. This freed up time for people whom didn't want to invest as much time in farming to do other activities.

Around the same time, as hundreds-of-thousands of people migrated to America, mothers were encouraged to set aside the cultural foods of their native home, which they were used to, in favor of 'convenience' foods that the Food Manufacturers of America were promoting at early as the 1800's, *with the intent to increase the consumer-base, of processed foods.*

America went from eating fresh food being produced by 90% of the population, with quality as the primary objective to 2% of the population controlling the entire food market, with control of the market and profit and long shelf life being the primary objectives, versus health-optimization and nutrition-density.

The results are that what is labeled food today is easier to get, easier to heat, faster, there are massive quantities available, it's very convenient, there are greater variety (a store where I shop has 40,000 different products), and it is cheaper to produce than ever.

Some of the results are that fiber is dramatically decreased, good sugars and fats are decreased, unhealthy sugars are increased, unhealthy fats are increased, salt is increased, fake foods, fats and sweeteners are added, toxins that excite the brain and central nervous system and starve the cells of health are added in, **so that as nutritional-deficiency proceeds, there's a sensory payoff/biochemical stimulus,** within the brain and nervous system.

Profit for the mass food producers has skyrocketed and so have the *de*-generative *dis*-eases! Profit for the food producers has skyrocketed while value for us consumers has plummeted, while little-by-little, the health of our nation is going downhill, resulting in the gross national product (money spent in America) accounts for 17% of every dollar spent…*meaning, the less nutrition people put in their body, the more is spent on healthcare!*

In fact, degenerative *dis*-eases are occurring at younger and younger ages. *Dis*-eases that used to be considered the aging process for 40-and-50-year-olds are showing up in people during their childhood, teen years, 20's-and-30's, now in record-breaking levels.

Fiber for instance:

Let's simplify this 'food processing' idea for a moment. If the only downside of processing our food was the fiber being removed, that alone has a significant impact on our ability to look and feel our best, as well as prevent *dis*-ease.

Fiber is simply the part of plants that is indigestible. In most cases, it doesn't get broken down much within our digestive system. It doesn't do anything to (directly) "make" more energy for activity, but the result of being clean on the inside, makes it easier for the body to produce energy and for other processes of the body to occur quicker.

Adults need to work up to eating about 50-grams of fiber each day. That is enough to fill about ⅓ of a sandwich-size plastic bag. Processed food has very little fiber at all. The average person whom is not counting how much they are getting consumes only about 8-to-12 grams each day. That is not enough.

Consider these things. Some surveys show that since the 1870's there has been a 90% decrease in the intake of fiber, among Americans. Fiber cleans the intestine from the inside out, preventing food and toxins from rotting in the gut, maintain blood sugar/energy levels as well as cholesterol levels.

Where might the people whom began eating less of the good stuff be 20-to-40 years later?

By 1910, Americans were eating 50% less Whole-foods like grains, beans, fresh fruits and vegetables. Hint, hint...this was before mass advertising kicked in to get people to eat the junky, empty, life-sapping processed stuff, in combination with eating less of the stuff that actually builds health, from the inside out one-cell-at-a-time (B.N.B.B.s). This was before television had the opportunity to convince children what would make them feel good to eat and at the same time starve their bodies into *de*-generative *dis*-ease like diabetes...***feeling full, but actually malnourished***...the same as being overweight or carrying an unhealthy amount of fat.

Oh, here they are...from 1931-to-1976 the occurrence of heart *dis*-ease jumped 800%.

Here are some others...from 1950-to-1996 people age 50-to-60 experienced a 44% increase in the rate of cancer. Prostate cancer jumped 100%. Breast cancer jumped 60%. Lung cancer increased 262%. It's to the point now that experts say every man will experience prostate cancer if something else doesn't kill him first...*inevitable, if we live long enough?*

Countries with a high intake of fiber in their diet, like Nigeria and Uganda, experience hundreds and literally thousands-of-times-less incidence of colon cancer.

Remember? Fiber cleans us from the inside out. There are many toxins in the environment, toxins our body produces as a result of being alive and fiber speeds the rate at which these toxins move through the body and prevents them from being re-absorbed and re-circulated into the system.

There was an article in the September 1987 issue of *Journal of the American Dietetic Association* entitled, *Fiber and colon cancer.* The authors summarized 40-different studies. Dr. Peter Greewald of The National Cancer Institute concluded that, *"...the association between high-fiber intake and lower-risk of cancer is consistent, coherent and strong."*

The body is designed to be like a fast-flowing, beautiful, clean stream. If we don't eat enough fiber, it becomes more like a swamp and it is directly reflected in the way we look, feel and perform. Toxins can build up in the body and the way they manifest as health problems is as varied as our fingerprints.

A study done by one of the most well-respected and renowned nutrition research companies demonstrated that the simple act of eating 15-grams, of fiber per day, (a very little bit), increases the rate at which stuff passes through the body by 45%. That means instead of being a swamp, the body becomes a fast-flowing stream, able to keep itself clean from the inside out.

Believe it or not, I have heard medical professionals whom don't believe that making toxins move through the faster has any bearing on optimal health and performance and they will even ignore the positive benefits their patients' experience when it doesn't match what they learned in medical school or what the prescription drug sales representatives promote. But, at the same time, health professionals see a lot of patients in the E.R. whom are severely constipated, from lacking adequate water and fiber intake (fruits and vegetables). What people don't seem to get is that you can get so constipated that surgery is out of the question. At a certain point, it becomes too dangerous to do surgery, since all that constipated material increases the risk of systemic infection. People do die this way.

The conditions that make sensible-supplementation of the B.N.B.B.s to your daily routine to conveniently make up for not even getting minimal amounts of government standards include:

- Increased salt,

- Increased bad fats,

- Increased fake fats,

- Increased simple sugars,

- Increased synthetic sweetners,

- Increased profit for companies,

- Increased tasty, chemicals (excito-toxins) and

- Decreased complex sugars, fiber and good fats.

Reason 44. Stuff called food really is not food at all:

The changes in the quality of our health and performance occur so slowly, we may not easily recognize what's happening. If overnight all the fresh food was replaced by fake food, so the producers could make lots of it, and within a week or two everyone began getting sick things would be different. It took me 15-years to notice that excessive sugar had any association with having a chronic sore throat. Much of what is happening with the food in America would be considered terrorism if it were being done by a different country. In essence, it is cellular terrorism. To those of us whom weren't alive 100-years ago, there is no way for us to know this or put the pieces together. A combination of factors for slow, gradual, socially acceptable, societal-genocide. *"As long as it occurs slow enough, we will let you stay in business because we make so much tax money from you and we don't want your lobbyists coming after us."*

The ability of nutritional-deficiencies to affect the body, even the genes of the body through soil depletion, over processed foods, excessive sugar and bad fats and even malnourishment through overfeeding starvation was recognized at least as early as the 1800's.

In 1939 Weston Price, D.D.S., published his monumental studies on world nutrition in his book, *Nutrition and Physical Degeneration*. There seem to be many critics of his work as there is for many whistle-blowers. Dr. Price traveled around the world documenting, through photography, the destruction of primitive cultures. He graphically caught the destruction occurring as indigenous cultures began adopting the eating habits, which I refer to as S.A.D.C.R.A.P. (Standard American Diet of Continuously & Repetitively Advertised Products), especially refined sugar.

As soon as the parents in the indigenous cultures began eating S.A.D.C.R.A.P. [they passed previously latent, inferior genetic traits to the very next generation] of children and *dis*-eases that had previously been latent, were now active *dis*-ease.

Peoples whom had a history of longevity and health, without *de*-generation, began breaking down within one-generation. People whom didn't have health problems, even though they had the genetic predispositions began experiencing what, in America, is referred to as hereditary *de*-generative *dis*-ease. Since history began, the indigenous people seemed to carry the *potential* for health susceptibilities like dental cavities. But they didn't manifest until processed foods were introduced into their diets.

As of 1992 there were about 400 different pesticides registered for use on American crops.

72 of them are classified as potential cancer-causing chemicals by the Environmental Protection Agency (EPA).

The Food and Drug Administration (FDA) inspects only about 2% of imported fruit and vegetables and this doesn't take into account genetically-modified organisms/foods (GMOs) which are banned in many countries due to how fast people and animals get systemically-ill as they are introduced into the food-chain or even the handling of GMO farming practices destroy those farmers' health.

The Department of Agriculture has found about 150 different chemicals in poultry and meat they analyzed.

More than 85,000 different chemicals have been introduced, in our environment, since the 1940's.

1,500 new chemicals are developed each year. About ½ are in common use today.

Less than 1,000 have been tested to definitively rule out if they cause cancer, let alone what they do to the body in combination with each other or their allergic, inflammatory and/or oxidative potential.

We have more chemicals in our environment now than any other time in recorded history. So much so it's difficult to avoid them. Poisons such as drugs, fertilizers, herbicides, pesticides and all the others break down or get 'detoxified' in the body in similar ways. During the detoxification process a literal free radical factory is established in the body releasing free radicals on a massive scale.

Chemical companies literally make new chemicals, then make up ways to get rid of them and get paid for them. They get us to put them in and on our food. Take them as drugs. Put them on our body. Put them in our air and water. Apply them to the grounds around our home. And apply them in our homes as 'cleaners'. The commercials and sales ads are so convincing, aren't they?

Only 10% of the things considered household products (like furniture polished, laundry products, dish cleanser, air fresheners and things of that nature), are tested for safety and few if any are tested in combination with each other.

People literally pay to have poisons in their home because the chemicals are labeled as cleaners. I have known people to 'clean' their homes with some of the most toxic products known because they associate the smell of the product as clean, even though they are toxic.

Dr. Bernard Jensen, author of, *Empty Harvest*, wrote, *"Also aware of this relationship was my late friend, J. I. Rodale of the Rodale Natural Foods Publishing empire. He often said he believed there was a correlation in the fact that my ancestral home of Denmark boasted two dubious records: Number one in both its use of artificial-fertilizers and its annual suicide rate. Rodale said he felt there was a direct correlation between Denmark's dead soil and its dead people."*

From 1947-to-1960 (era of surplus of the World War II chemicals), pesticide production increased from 259,000 pounds per year to over 6,000,000 pounds…instead of simply using up the bomb-making materials as fertilizer, it started a whole new industry…this came about from noticing that where the bombs were deployed, the grass grew faster!

In 1948, Paul Miller of Switzerland won a Nobel Prize for his discovery of chlorophenathane, dichlorodiphenyltrichlorethane. Sounds like it would be safe to test on people, right? Its common name is DDT. One of the most deadly, cancer-causing pesticides known.

By the 1960's D.D.T. was banned from use in the United States. It has been found everywhere on the planet. Even in fish and wildlife, where it was never even used. Penguins at the North Pole have it in their bodies. It has been found in all food and drink. It has contaminated the Earth, the food-chain and people. It doesn't go away. It sticks in the fat of the body.

Get this:

D.D.T. is banned in the U.S. but it is still manufactured, used outside the U.S. in other countries where the people don't know the danger. Then the food is imported back into the U.S. and sold to us at the grocery store. D.D.T. is a completely human-manufactured molecule. Nature can't break it down, under usual circumstances. It can reside in full-toxicity for thousands-of-years, in the water and soil.

When I was managing the produce department at a grocery-store, I began to notice all kinds of warning labels on the produce boxes that the fruits and vegetables are delivered in. One-by-one, I saved the warning labels. Mostly out of curiosity. One day, I decided to research what the ingredients were, so I got on the net. The following are a few of the actual ingredients that you ingest if you eat non-organic produce, along with the primary warnings issued by the EPA. When you attend one of my group presentations, you can see the display of labels for yourself. I call it the *"Wall of Death"*. Here's some of them that are still used today:

Iprodione:

Fungicide; hazard: taken orally, on skin, in eyes, inhaled. Dangerous to the environment, children, humans, domestic animals, livestock and other.

Triforine:

Fungicide for mildew and molds; hazard: irritant, can decrease food intake, decrease in body weight, decrease in pregnancy, increase in resorption of fetus, adverse effects on red blood cells and chemical pneumenitis.

Breakdown in surface water – no information available.

Vegitation takes it up through the roots – phytotoxic to pears.

DCNA:

Fungicide; hazard: oral, skin, eye, can cause skin reaction and hazard to inhale. Dangerous to the environment, water, fish, children, humans and drift.

Sodium O-Phenylphenate:

Fungicide; hazard: oral, eye, fatal if swallowed, corrosive. Used as a wash, soak and dip.

Chlorpropham:

Pesticide; hazard: oral, eye, skin, inhaled, growth regulator, fatal if swallowed.

Diphenyamine:

Fungicide; hazard:oral, eye, skin. Used as a wash, soak and dip.

The next one I was really curious about, since I recognized the name, but I couldn't place it. I used to be a horse veterinary assistant. Almost every day we treated horses for worm infestation…bananans have horse wormer applied to them.

Thiabenadazole – Mintezol®:

May cause dry mouth, dry eyes, dry nose, liver problems, kidney problems, drowsiness, avoid driving, operating machinery. If you experience any of the following, call your physician: blurred vision, yellow vision, skin rash, hives, red peeling skin, fever, chills, dark urine, seizures, jaundice, bad odor of urine, ringing in ears, flushing of skin. Anthelmintic; treats worm infections, will not prevent worm infections.

Sodium Orthopenylphenol:

Fungicide: Cresylic Acid.

Imazil and Orthophenylphenate:

Fungicides – Florida Department of Citrus; Anti-mold agent.

All of these are just a sampling of the chemicals applied to conventiaonlly farmed produce.

Toxic behavioral changes:

A friend of a friend of mine had a client with a five-year old son whom was in the doctor's office more than once-a-month, with allergy and asthma problems. The mother of the boy changed brands of laundry detergent to a safe, non-toxic type. Her son's asthma and allergies went away.

I know of another parent whom did the same thing. Her son's health and behavior problems simply went away. Then mom forgot why she had quit using the conventional laundry and 'cleaning' products. She cleaned her home and when her little boy came home, he first started behaving kind of strange and it escalated into violent behavior, running, almost flying around the home screaming. She remembered how much better he was months earlier. She re-cleaned all the surfaces with the safe, non-toxic cleaners and her son calmed down right before her eyes.

Back in 1993 when I first began putting all the pieces together, I completely changed brands and converted my home to a non-toxic home. I got rid of everything in my apartment that you can purchased in the 'sneeze-and-wheeze-aisle' of your favorite grocery store. My health improved dramatically, relatively quickly.

You might not be aware of it yet, but all the different products you use in your home to clean with leaves residue. On your towels, on your wash clothes, on the sheets, blankets and pillowcases. All, of these things, add to the work-load of the body attempting to detoxify the stuff from the body. If you haven't been aware of this yet, it might seem like such a small detail it could not possibly have an impact on you or your family's health, especially so when you have been skipping the B.N.B.B.s. But when you do switch over, you'll know for yourself. The safe, non-toxic cleaners sometimes cost more up front. That's because they're made out of natural-resources, like plant extracts and oils, whereas the commercial ones are made mostly out of inexpensive, petroleum by-products...*the leftovers from the production of gasoline.*

The same stuff left over after making gasoline and oil being used to make synthetic vitamins and personal care products...*hmmm*. These products seriously affect the nervous, respiratory and immune system. Just like super-size fast-food meals, they are practically giving the stuff away now, and if your priority is other than optimal health and performance, the money you save at the cash register is a reflection of how much value you place on your health.

When I changed brands, it took about five-washings to get the residue from the toxic stuff out of my laundry. All that stuff goes onto the skin, is absorbed and then has to be filtered and cleansed out of the body by the internal organs.

On March 22, 2001 a Seattle Newspaper ran an article entitled, *"We are walking, talking waste sites."*

It seems the Federal Centers for Disease Control and Prevention did a study in an attempt to measure pollution in human bodies. It's well-known that mosquito insecticide used heavily over 30-years, hasn't diluted in the environment anymore. D.D.T. never biodegrades down. It's a cancerous chemical and the government said it was completely safe as the neighborhoods around Seattle were showered with the stuff as children played outside.

In this new study, the CDC reported finding high levels of toxins in common, everyday personal care and household products, like soap and shampoo. Makes sense, right? You want to get clean, so you lather up and shower off with a handful of toxins?

These chemicals known as phthalates have been shown for more than 20-years to cause birth defects in the male sex organs as well as low sperm count and atrophy of the male sex organs. The phthalates also seemed to change the female development hormones in girls.

Blood and urine samples were taken from 3,800 people in 1999 also found evidence of widespread pesticide contamination because people are being exposed to more pesticides than the government group previously thought.

10% of children and women had dangerously high levels of heavy metals that are toxic to the nervous system and reproductive system especially.

The study tested for 27-toxic-substances commonly found in cosmetics, soaps, hair care products and baby pacifiers. Does this make sense? Poisonous chemicals in the stuff we put on our skin and in baby's moths to pacify them, because they can and mostly because it's a buyer-beware market.

All the women and children tested had these poisonous chemicals in their bodies. Some environmental and public health groups have called for a ban on these toxic-substances, but the National Toxicology Program – a federal task force – recommended against a ban.

...in other words,

Sandra Tiery, spokesperson for The American Chemistry Council (a chemical industry trade association) responded to the CDCP's study saying, *"Data alone is not an indication that anybody's health is being impaired...the health significance."* Whaaat?

The CDC plans to eventually expand its surveys to 100-toxic-substances of the 85,000 than have been manufactured, since World War II.

In other words, *"I'm being paid to talk, talk, talk and tie this thing up in red tape for at least the next 10-years, so we can make a trillion dollars from using this stuff, we have more money to spend on this than you ever will because you're funded by tax-dollars and we are being paid by consumers whom by our products, without knowing the danger,"...if I did not argue this point and talk in circles I wouldn't be able to pay off my college debt...we already burned the proof of danger," ...blah, blah, blah."*

In other words, people, it's up to each person to learn which companies make a profit by improving health/building health and which ones make a profit without a philosophy other than promoting products as safe when they are actually harmful...simply put, it's a buyer-beware market.

The government agencies do not have the financial resources nor the people-power to test all the 85,000 different chemicals by themselves, let alone in combination, nor their effects on health. WHAT THAT MEANS is the process of creating health-building products and products that are non-toxic is left to the manufacturers themselves! That means buying products that are guaranteed to be non-toxic! You get to choose the business and operating philosophy of the company you give your money to...and your health improves dramatically as a result.

Companies don't have to prove their products are safe to sell them. Even when people begin getting sick it can take 10-to-100 years to get the product banned because the government has to prove the danger because trade associations (groups of business people lose money when their poisonous products are banned) lobby to prevent the public from knowing what's in their products and the effects their products have on health

. In a lot of cases, chemicals that are banned or limited in their use due to health danger (as one kind of product), can be promoted and sold openly labeled as a different product. **In other words, some chemicals that are considered dangerous to handle are added to dietary-supplements, skin care products and personal care products because the rules which apply to one kind of product (say, a yard care products), don't carry over to other classes of products.**

It's this combination of chemicals and lack of nutrition-density, to maintain that body, that is causing widespread as well as un-diagnosable, man-made health conditions that aren't easily recognizable nor diagnosable, as well as epidemic levels of obesity and weight gain.

https://blog.bulletproof.com posted, *Why Getting Your Nutrition Only from Food is A Bad Idea:*

As the Standard American Diet (SAD) shifts further and further away from nutrient-dense foods like high-quality animal protein and vegetables, nutrient-deficiency is becoming a widespread epidemic. But even if you're following a more nutrient-dense diet full of quality protein and fats, you can no longer rely on getting all of your nutrients from food. Nutrient-deficiencies hurt your performance, causing DNA damage, making you age faster, and contributing to chronic *dis*-ease. If that's not convincing enough, here are 10-more reasons you should consider nutrient supplementation.

10 Reasons You Should Take Supplements by blog.bulletproof.com.

1.You eat a Standard American Diet (S.A.D.):

Grains, legumes, and most forms of modern dairy are not food. The purpose of consuming food is to nourish the body and mind. These foods do the opposite.

First of all, grains, legumes, and conventional dairy are low in nutrients and difficult for a lot of people to digest. Grains and legumes contain phytic acid and other compounds that can interfere with nutrient absorption and can cause intestinal damage, which makes it even harder for your body to absorb nutrients. Even if you've stopped eating these foods, you may be in nutrient debt or have lingering intestinal damage, which is interfering with nutrient absorption. Dairy, especially conventional dairy, is inflammatory and difficult to digest for many people. It also contains mycotoxins which are extremely inflammatory.

2. Soil depletion:

Improper farming practices deplete the soil of essential-nutrients. When plants are repeatedly grown on the same land, the soil loses vitamins, minerals, and microbes faster than they can be replaced. Over time, the plants have fewer nutrients to grow.

Fertilizer contains just enough nutrition for the plant to survive until harvesting, but not enough to support human health. In addition, most plants are not harvested fresh. They sit on trucks, shelves, and counters for weeks before being eaten. Over time, the nutrient content of these plants decreases.

Most modern fruits and vegetables are grown (to increase their sugar content), not their nutrient-density value. As a result, the most common fruits and vegetables are artificially high in fructose and **lower in key-nutrients, before we even purchase them.**

When plants contain fewer nutrients, the mammals whom eat these plants can also become malnourished. A study published in the *Journal of Nutrition and Health* found copper levels in the UK have dropped 90% in dairy, 55% in meat, and 76% in vegetables. Copper is an essential-nutrient that helps to regulate several pathways in the body, including energy production and brain function.

3. Water depletion:

Water is also depleted of minerals due to modern production methods. There is a huge variation in the mineral content of bottled and tap water, with tap water generally having more. Most water filters remove important minerals such as Magnesium, which is essential for more than 300-biochemical-reactions, in the body. Up until recently, clean, unfiltered fresh water was the main source of Magnesium for humans. Not anymore. Our water is filtered of essential minerals like Magnesium, contaminated with chlorine, and fortified with potentially harmful chemicals like fluoride.

The filtration of precious minerals from water could explain why people whom drink water higher in Calcium than Magnesium, develop more myocardial infarcts and ischemic heart *dis*-ease.

4. Low-calorie diets are low-nutrient diets:

I know this is a crazy idea, but starving yourself of key-nutrients is bad. Consuming a low-calorie diet means you're consuming less nutrition-density. As humans, we're designed to consume larger amounts of nutrient-dense calories to meet our body's needs. When you're constantly restricting your caloric-intake, it's easy to become malnourished. When you're consuming low-quality foods, like pasteurized non-fat milk and other 'Franken-foods' you have to eat *even more* to obtain the right amounts of nutrition. That's how you get fat. And just one more example of why food quality matters…calories consumption is increasing, but nutrition-density is inherently decreasing…***filled up, but empty.***

Animal-based-foods are generally higher in calories and nutrients, so it's no surprise that's where the majority of calories came from in early human development. Since the modern trend is to reduce the consumption of animal-based-foods, people are consuming fewer nutrients, per unit of food…***empty-filler***

5. Non-organic foods contain fewer nutrients:

Non-Certified-Organically grown, pesticide-treated vegetables generally are lower in cancer-fighting polyphenols than Certified-Organically-Grown foods. This is because the plant produces polyphenols as a defense against bugs and pathogens. When there is no reason to defend themselves, the plant stops producing polyphenols and your body and brain suffer the consequences.

There is also evidence that glyphosate – RoundUp™ herbicide – chelates minerals in crops on which it is sprayed…in other words, it holds the nutrients in the soil rather than allowing them to be taken up by the plants themselves. It remains to be seen how much of an impact this effect has, but it's safe to avoid GMO foods for a variety of other reasons.

Unfortunately, Certified-Organically-Grown is not always possible, due to financial or logistical reasons. Even when you can find Certified-Organically-Grown foods, they aren't necessarily better. Certified-Organically-Grown relates to the purity of the plants [until the time of harvest], whereas the B.N.B.B.s, as I refer to them, are checked and double-checked, even after manufacturing for impurities…so, they are cleaner than what we know as Certified-Organic-Foods…*as it should be.*

6. Grain-fed meat & cooked/conventional dairy:

Compared to grass-fed meat, grain-fed meat is abysmally low in antioxidants, micronutrients, fatty acids, minerals, and vitamins. Grains are not a food for humans or grazing animals. When herbivores are fed grains, they become malnourished, just like humans….**fat but mal-nourished.** Grain-fed meat and farmed seafood can also serve as a carrier for more toxins, which increases nutrient needs.

Raw, unpasteurized, unprocessed, full-fat dairy can be good for you, but the kind most people buy at the grocery store is not ok. The majority of nutrients in milk are found in the fat (cream). When you remove or reduce the fat, you are removing and reducing the nutrient content. Pasteurization destroys some of the nutrients in both skim and full-fat milk. Conventionally-farmed dairy is also high in aflatoxin and other mycotoxins that were in the cattle's feed.

7. Toxin exposure:

Your body needs nutrients to deal with toxins. When more toxins are present, you need more nutrients. If you're living in a cave or the Garden of Eden, this will be less of a concern. If you're like the rest of us mortals – you're exposed to a litany of toxins, on a daily basis.

Here are just some of the things your body has to contend with:

● Food toxins,

● Unnatural lighting,

● Stress and lack of sleep,

● Industrial solvents and cleaners and

● Xenoestrogens (plastics, BPA, some molds, petroleum products).

There are hundreds-of-other-sources, of unnatural stress that increase the body's need for proper nutrition. Even if you're doing everything right in terms of diet – *it's almost impossible to get all of your nutrients from food alone, consistently enough to make a difference.*

Our bodies weren't designed to deal with these toxins using only nutrition from food. Instead, it's good to support detox and methylation pathways* with supplements.

*The Methylation Pathway. Methylation is the process of controlled transfer of a methyl group (one carbon atom and three hydrogen atoms) onto amino acids, proteins, enzymes, and DNA in every cell and tissue of the body to *regulate healing, cell energy, genetic expression of DNA, neurological function, liver detoxification, immunity, etc.*

8. Nutrient-absorption declines with age:

Several studies have shown kids need more nutrients to support growth, and older people need more nutrients due to malabsorption. As you age, hydrochloric acid and digestive enzyme production naturally declines, making it difficult for you to break down and absorb nutrients from your foods. As you age, you also often begin taking medications which can interfere with nutrient absorption. This means you need to take more nutrients in the most absorbable form possible. *The B.N.B.B.s fill in all these gaps.*

9. Exercise increases nutrient needs:

Athletes often think tons of exercise is the key to a long and healthy life (it's not). They are among the first to denounce supplementation as unnecessary, often with the idea that exercise is the best medicine. I don't advocate high amounts of exercise, but this is an important point: *If you're doing exercise which substantially depletes energy reserves, you're also using more nutrients for energy production and recovery.* As a result, athletes are at an even higher risk of nutrient deficiencies. Since many athletes eat a low nutrient, high toxin diet – this is a serious concern.

10. Supplementation may help you live longer:

Aging is a natural process, but it's not fun. If there are supplements that can delay this process, why not take them? As long as there isn't an undue risk of harm, it's hard to justify avoiding a substance simply because our ancestors didn't have access to it. There is good reason to believe a higher intake of nutrients may prolong life. Our hunter-gatherer ancestors may have been malnourished, at certain times, which is not beneficial. If supplements can buy you a few more years of quality life, why not take them?

11. Expense & health:

Whether we like it or not, sometimes supplements are cheaper than real food. In the case of something like salmon, it may be better for you to supplement with a high-quality fish or krill oil than to settle for a farmed-variety. Farmed-salmon is low in Omega-3's (good fats) and higher in toxins.

Farmed-salmon are higher in parasites and bacteria. In order to hide the sickly appearance of farmed salmon meat, the fish are fed a pink pigment to change their tissue color. Farmed-salmon contains 16-times more PCB's and pesticides than wild. Wild-salmon is often more expensive than grass-fed beef and presents more of a health risk than benefit. Grass-fed beef has enough Omega-3's by itself, but supplementation may be a good idea for some people (like kids, adults, athletes and seniors).

The idea that you can get all your nutrients from food is fine in theory, but virtually impossible in practice. Soil and water depletion, food and environmental toxins, poor absorption, pesticides, exercise, and lack of calories can all cause nutrient deficiencies. There is evidence that consuming nutrients from food is more beneficial than supplements, which is why you should focus on a nutrient-rich diet first, as the foundation. However, it's rarely enough anymore, so back up your Whole-foods with the B.N.B.B.s!

Chapter Eight

The sun will come out tomorrow…

Reason 45. Live in a climate where you don't get enough sunlight?

We get Vitamin D from sunlight, from certain foods and from dietary-supplements.

Unfortunately, most people don't eat enough good food to get enough Vitamin D from food to meet the demands of their body. Secondly, a lot of people don't live in a climate where we get enough sunlight to produce enough Vitamin D in the skin. Supplementation is a reliable way to get a consistent, safe level of Vitamin D, which supports healthy bones and other health processes, thereby preventing osteopenia and osteoporosis, depression and many other health symptoms.

Many internal medicine physicians are now testing all their patients' level of Vitamin D and finding that most people are deficient, unless they have been supplementing, with the B.N.B.B.s for some time.

A common problem I see nowadays, is people whom acknowledge the benefit and importance of dietary-supplementation, but do not realize the importance or distinction of food concentrates vs synthetic (prescription or pharmaceutical-grade), and crystalline or extracted (food-based or vegetarian-formulas).

The latter two do not produce adequate blood levels nor the benefits of improved bone mass and immune support. I have heard of people taking what would be considered toxic level of Vitamin D only to find that their blood levels aren't increasing and even decreasing.

As long as someone won't acknowledge there is a difference, in the "types" of dietary-supplements, they are likely to continue doing what isn't working and wonder why their blood plasma levels aren't increasing and why their bones aren't reflecting the increased consumption of the supplement. They may think of themselves as a special-case or that it is a medical-mystery…and it is to those whom won't feed their cells with real nutrition. It's sad. All I can do is deliver the message and I can't help everyone.

Once someone is so depleted that their bones are showing signs of *de*-generation, e.g. osteoporosis, osteopenia and fractures, if they won't do the very action I'm suggesting there isn't anything else I can do for them because at that point it's about them and their daily lifestyle habits…the very best physicians in the world can't medicate a person enough to make up for what they are purposely withholding nutritionally from their body, on a daily basis. I knew a man that ate only one-meal-a-day, for decades and to his surprise several of his vertebra fractured from lack of nutritional-density…he was a physician whom was the medical director of an HMO. He couldn't understand that nutrition has to be put in the body (consumed), nor that one-meal-per-day, without supplements, was adequate to preserve his nutrition-surplus.

Dr. Catherine Northrup, MD, author of *Women's Bodies Women's Minds,* says the RDA of 400 units/day of Vitamin D is too low and that 2000 units of Vitamin D is more appropriate.

A 'big-picture' priority point here regarding Vitamin D and its optimal absorption and assimilation into stronger, healthier bone density is the synergistic relationship of Vitamin D and ***all the other*** vitamins, minerals and nutritional-factors (both named and unnamed). A common, big mistake the majority of consumers make is to think in terms of chasing symptoms with individual nutrients, for examples:

- B12 for energy,

- Iron for anemia,

- Niacin for high cholesterol,

- Vitamin D & Calcium for bones and

- Folate for prevention of birth defects.

and the list goes on…

The relationship of Calcium and Vitamin D for healthy bones and the consequential supplementing of the two is short-sighted and symptom-chasing mentality, indicative of a bigger, much broader underlying problem of wide-spectrum deficiency, of the B.N.B.B.s.

Here's what I mean by that: No body part or system is dependent on any (single) B.N.B.B. for its health and integrity. Each part and system of the body is dependent on *all* the B.N.B.B.s and supplementing with only a couple or even a few of the B.N.B.B.s often is reflected in little to no improvement in the person's symptoms and/or health and performance.

For example; a person with low bone-density or any of the other bone problems, nowadays, may take extra Vitamin D and Calcium, but the bones as biologically active organs and systems require *all* the B.N.B.B.s, so they likely will not respond optimally or at all, by chasing symptoms with one vitamin or mineral.

Each system of the body requires **all** the B.N.B.B.s, as we can't calculate all the ways the B.N.B.B.s interact, depend and interrelate to one another, to make up this machine we call the body. Supplementing with individual nutrients, without broad-spectrum nutritional coverage of all the body's requirements, *as a starting point* is simply addressing what *is* known, not what isn't known. And what is known doesn't even begin to utilize the massive complexity of what we refer to as nature.

Think about it.

Take *all* 7 of the B.N.B.B.s and you'll be a lot further ahead… you'll notice the difference in the way you feel and in the results of your clinical blood tests and the results of your bone-density tests.

Reason 46. Anemia:

This one is a little self-explanatory, but the point is that if you are anemic, that means you aren't eating enough nutrition to meet the demands of your body. *So much so that it is showing up on blood screenings.*

Anemia most often refers to not having enough Iron in the blood, but it points to the idea that if you don't have enough Iron (one mineral that is common in food), you're likely short on other ones as well, it's just more common to test for Iron than the others. Some nutrients are considered to be produced within the body of healthy individuals (like some of the B vitamins), the question to me again is the relative term 'healthy'. Either from too little good, Whole-food or because your activity level is high enough that your body is using more nutrition than you are putting back in, the body begins getting so deficient of the B.N.B.B.s that it shows up in the way you look and feel (pale, tired and difficulty concentrating).

Many children in America are anemic upon entering school for the first time. Women and anyone whom loses blood are susceptible as well as athletes. I heard of one of the top cross-country runners here in Washington State a couple-years back. He was an amazing runner and consistently blew away all the competition. He ran about 40-miles a week, which would lead one to imagine he was a healthy individual, but alike a lot of people they think that because they are gifted or have natural ability they can skip the nutrition part...*that's because they can get away without supplementing longer than they should.* Long story short, he described how one day, when he was running, he felt like he, *"...hit a wall."* His energy level dropped off and he couldn't run anymore. He felt light headed, dizzy and weak.

In other words, he had used up so much of at least some of the Basic Nutritional Building Blocks, in his body that his blood couldn't carry enough oxygen anymore (anemia).

A main point here: ***Just because you can, doesn't mean you should.*** If you really want to perform your best, whether you are a stay-at-home-mom or a medical-school-student or a professional-athlete, make sure you have a surplus of the B.N.B.B.s.

On September 2, 2008 Matt Lauer, NBC reporter reported that a one-cent increase in the price of milk increases the cost of milk for school lunch budgets by $54,000,000.00. *per year*...get it? The current nutrition standards are also based on saving money, as a higher priority than health. ***The financial responsibility is passed on to consumers whom want better health than what minimum recommendations would provide...have to do it yourself!***

Reason 47. Vegan or Vegetarian:

Anyone whom lives a vegetarian lifestyle has every right to eat or not eat whatever they want. That's one of the benefits of living in America.

The way I look at it, friends, after four-decades of experimenting with food and nutrition, is that a clean-diet reduces the level of toxins entering the body, but the B.N.B.B. s make up for what the diet is missing. Its not as simple as trying to eliminate S.A.D.C.R.A.P.

Think about it, folks. The RDA and DVI%s, as well as the food guide pyramid and other government guidelines, are designed around an average human person getting 2,000 calories a day and yet, we have seen athletes eating 14,000 calories a day and even then [they are deficient of at least some of the key nutrients leaving them vulnerable to all the *de*-generative *dis*-eases] that all the other people whom aren't eating near that amount of food each day. Yes, these are competitive athletes, but never the less, even at that amount of food they were still deficient of some nutrients. The 2,000 calories a day guideline for the average person is, in my professional opinion, banking on the fact that the average person won't be active enough to use up the minimum amount of nutrition they supposedly have...a set up for a nation of overweight, unhealthy people that gets worse with each successive generation.

If they aren't getting enough nutrition, *whom is?*

Thinking, believing and saying you eat balanced does not equate to having enough nutrition in your bloodstream, available to your cells in real time on a day to day basis.

Reason 48. Considering elective-surgery?

Going into surgery you want your nervous system to be prepared for the stress, your immune system prepared to resist potential infection (e.g. staph, MRSA and CDC), and the body in general to resist the shock and trauma of the surgery itself. You don't get this from eating three-square-meals-a-day. Supplementing with the B.N.B.B.s can provide a nutritional-cushion that the body needs to recover from surgery.

Stephan Chaney, MD Professor of Biophysics, Biochemistry and Nutrition at The North Carolina Medical School shared a study that he found. Conducted at the University of Toronto more than 20-years ago, demonstrated the effects of nutritional status of people whom had general elective surgery.

• 75% of those people with poor nutritional-status needed antibiotics and their hospital stay was an average of 48 days.

• 20% of those with excellent nutritional-status needed antibiotics and their average stay was 18 days, at a savings of $20,000.00. per patient.

The Western Journal of Medicine, 1997;166:306-312 reported that hospital costs in the U.S. alone could be reduced by $20,000,000,000.00 ($20-billion), a year, if people consumed, what I refer to as the B.N.B.B.s, *daily.*

Adrianne Bendich, PhD, and her collaborators analyzed hospital charges for just three preventable *dis*-eases: *birth defects, low-weight, premature births and heart dis-ease.* The researchers calculated that hospital charges for these here conditions could be reduced by 40%, 60% and 38% respectively. The cost of the dietary-supplementation of the B.N.B.B.s is substantially lower than the cost of hospital care. At the same time I talk to people all the time that feel if someone else won't pay for their B.N.B.B.s they're not going to take them. Crazy!

Reason 49. Considering mandatory surgery?

See #48

Reason 50. Preparing for surgery?

See #48

Reason 51. Recovering from surgery?

See #48

Reason 52. Old enough to get pregnant?

One of the biggest oversights, in regard to supplementation, of the B.N.B.B.s is that just because you aren't *planning* on getting pregnant you don't need to think about the nutritional-needs of a fetus. The potential of getting pregnant is enough reason to take them.

Unfortunately, this is one of those cases where the B.N.B.B.s have to be on board **ahead of time.** The new baby has specific requirements, especially during the first-trimester of pregnancy, when women often don't know they are pregnant. During this time, critical windows of growth and development are taking place that affect the baby for the rest of his/her life. Birth defects are one of those preventable health conditions that can turn out as a beautiful thing or a devastating over sight.

So, the point is whether you are old enough to get pregnant, not whether you are planning to get pregnant. As you know, many babies come into this world unplanned. And if mom doesn't have enough nutrition in her body for herself where is baby supposed to get it? ***Nutrition doesn't appear in the body out of thin air!***

If you're old enough to get pregnant you need the B.N.B.B.s to protect the unexpected baby leading up to and during the first-trimester of pregnancy, *when the nervous system of the baby requires nutrition-density to develop without neural tube defects.*

53. Upper-brain/Pre-frontal cortex:

This is the part of the nervous system that has the most to do with mental clarity, mental stamina, learning new things, getting along well in relationships, making good decisions, taking action based on your goals and more importantly the ability of a person to lose weight, without having cravings and being able to sustain a fitness program…in other words, *'follow-through'.*

When the upper-brain is fueled, it's much easier to take consistent action, with regard to activities and lifestyle promoting long-term health, wellness and vitality...*carry out goals.* ***Finish things.***

Folks whom don't get enough B.N.B.B.s can seem depressed, apathetic, unmotivated, stuck in their feelings and as if they enjoy complaining without being able to follow through on actions suggested by their family, friends and medical-professionals…*while at the same time unaware of what is actually going on in their brain.*

Once a person eats and supplements in ways that feed and fuel the upper-brain they have the opportunity to contrast the difference between how they feel before and after. I think most people prefer feeling good, but most people don't know they needed (were needing) the B.N.B.B.s until they get enough of them to reflect on how much better they feel, *now.*

A pattern I have noticed over-the-(years is that people whom are the most deficient nutritionally) 'poo-poo' even the idea that nutrition may help them. There are real reasons for this confused perception, related to the front of the brain missing out on the nutrition the brain needs to recognize malnutrition! A Catch-22!

54. Cardiovascular system:

The body is constantly distributing and *re*-distributing the B.N.B.B. resources, that you put in your body, to maintain a nutritional-homeostasis.

We aren't born with enough nutrition to last our entire life, any more than a new car has enough fuel to last the life of the car.

When the muscles need Calcium and Vitamin D, where are they going to get them?..the muscles get them from the bones, of course. And that principle exists with each of the B.N.B.B.s, for the life of the individual.

If you think of a person whom says they don't *'buy into'* the idea of dietary-supplements and yet have a need for nutrition greater than what they eat, where is it that they aren't connecting the dots? At that point the real question is how to get the highest quality B.N.B.B.s.

In my experience, each and every system of the body require the B.N.B.B.s in order to keep themselves in good operating order and when the body doesn't have enough B.N.B.B.s the body seems to begin *de*-generating into *dis*-ease. The area of the body which suffers first, second and third depends on biological predispositions of the individual. But biology is not destiny and just like Dr. Weston Price's research showed, hereditary predispositions prompted by nutritional-apathy is just as reversible with consistent application. Even with addicts, brain scans show that lost gray matter in the front of the brain can be replaced, when health and lifestyle choices improve...*in other words, you can effectively rebuild the brain.*

In other words, your body requires the B.N.B.B.s, whether you are capable of 'conceiving' it at this time or not. Simply make a commitment to start and follow through for a-year-or-so. I think you'll be pleasantly surprised and if you find you just aren't worth the investment you can stop at any time and no harm done.

The B.N.B.B.s do not treat these conditions, but simply replace the fundamental building materials of the body structure itself. A side benefit is that as nature replenishes the heart tissue itself the structure, function and capability of the heart can normalize. Since the symptoms of the underlying scarcity are improved the symptoms seem to vacate and the original requirement for the medication also subsides unless the corresponding deficiency of the B.N.B.B.s is allowed to recur sufficiently, for the signs and symptoms to return.

Let's think about this whole heart *dis*-ease problem, for a minute:

In case you did not get it yet, a lot of heart *dis*-ease is preventable. Just like all the other *de*-generative *dis*-eases so common today in an over-fed under-nourished society, you can control many of the factors. Heart *dis*-ease, one of the number one killers in America and it takes 10-30 years to set-in, real good.

Along the way to death, people begin experiencing chest pains, shortness of breath, inability to move and take care of themselves, high cholesterol, lowered energy, decreased circulation to the fingers, toes, brain, eyes as well as the sexual organs begin to fail because blood, oxygen and nutrition cannot get to the when the blood vessels and arteries are all clogged up...*for eating chips and doughnuts*...**there's only so many hours in the day to get nutrition!**

Impotence and inability to have an orgasm are just the beginning. The drugs used to 'control' and 'manage' all the symptoms of eating and drinking too much of the wrong stuff can make the problems even worse.

If it were as simple as living your life to the extreme, eating, drinking and partying to the max and then you peacefully die in your sleep, or even instantly dropping dead, never knowing what hit you that would be one thing. But it's just not that easy. A lot of people just get severely injured from all that fast-energy and junk food. Then they have to live through even greater misery…to the point where they cannot even get out of bed to go to the bathroom.

With my own dad for instance, his arteries had hardened and became inflexible, which gave him severe chest pains, so bad he couldn't walk across the yard, because he was breathless and in so much pain. That is called angina pectoralis (pain in the chest). He had several pain attacks, every week. His doctor never told him what I'm going to gift you with.

Did you know?

• 2/3 the people whom have a heart attack die, within the first-hour of a heart attack.

• More women than men die this way.

• Heart *dis*-ease kills more women in America than the next 8-top killers combined.

• More African Americans than Caucasians die this way.

• For those that survive the first heart attack, within 6-months, 18% of men and 34% of women have a 2nd heart attack.

• For those that survive the first heart attack, within one-year, 25% of men and 38% of women have a 2nd heart attack.

• For those that survive the first heart attack, 8% of men and 11% of women have a stroke, which can cause paralysis.

• For those that survive the first heart attack, 22% of men and 46% of women are permanently disabled.

According to Dr. Michael Longo, MD, Deputy Chief of Cardiology Heart Institute of the Virginia Mason Medical Center, ***"Heart dis-ease kills more women than 6 times the number of all the cancers combined."***

"In 250,000 Americans, the first signs of heart dis-ease is sudden death and up to 50,000 of those people die at a very young age, like Ted Demme." Mr. Demme was a TV and film director, whom directed *Blow* and *Beautiful Girls* whom died at age 38 of a heart attack, from a condition known as sudden cardiac death, which afflicts thousands-of-Americans, each year.

Dr. Matthew Budoff, a Cardiologist at Harbor UCLA Medical Center, said the likely condition, *"...was a detectable disease that could have been treated before he suffered an early death."* Budoff said the young director probably had plaque building up in his arteries for years. *"It's a process that occurs over months or years and most likely occurs from a combination of genetic factors, plus cholesterol, plus high blood pressure."*

When the body is nutritionally-deficient, no amount of medicine will solve the problem.

So that's the bad news... here is the good news:

• Each 1% you reduce your cholesterol level you decrease your chance of heart attack by 2%.

• Lowering cholesterol level can actually halt the progress of heart *dis*-ease.

• Lifestyle changes, including eating for optimal health and exercising regularly can reverse the plaque buildup in the arteries, which is one of the main problems causing heart attack.

• Outward appearances are not an indicator of health. One of the greatest marathon runners of all time died of a massive heart attack during a run. He had the stereotypical runner's build (Jim Fixx).

Solutions:

Examples of studies which demonstrate how to dramatically reduce your risk of heart attack.

Study #1:

A supplemental combination of fiber and exercise, with a focus on body fat-loss, demonstrated an average drop in cholesterol levels, in four-weeks, of 15%, which reduces the risk of heart attack by 30%. This combination worked better than some of the cholesterol drugs, without the side-effects.

Study #2:

220 people were given 800 milligrams of garlic (about one small clove), for four-months. On average cholesterol levels dropped 12% (reduction of heart attack risk by 24%).

Study #3:

Performed at Munich University. A low-fat diet combined with garlic reduced cholesterol by 20% (reduction of heart attack risk by 40%).

Study #4:

Performed at University of Illinois. Susan Potter PhD found that isolated soy protein (25-50 grams), reduced cholesterol by 12% (reduction of heart attack risk by 24%).

Study #5:

Performed at Harvard University and published in *The New England Journal of Medicine*, Dr. Meir J Stampfer did a study on 87,000 female nurses. Those taking a Vitamin E supplement had a 30% reduction in the risk of heart attack or coronary heart *dis*-ease.

It is my understanding that Dr. Stapfer originally intended to prove Vitamin E had no benefit on preventing heart *dis*-ease. Dr. Stampfer was quoted as saying, *"It just did not seem plausible that a simple maneuver like taking Vitamin E would have such a profound effect."*

Study #6:

Performed at Harvard University on 46,000 male health professionals, over a four-year period. Those supplementing their Whole-foods with Vitamin E showed a 25% reduction in the risk of heart attack.

Study #7:

Performed at The Center for Human Nutrition at Southwestern Medical Center, in Dallas Texas, Dr. Ishwarlal Jialal published his results in the medical journal, *Arteriosclerosis, Thrombosis and Vascular Biology*. 48 men in a placebo-controlled and randomized study.

Vitamin E supplements were given in doses of 60, 200, 400, 800 and 1,200 international units each day. Bad cholesterol oxidation levels (LDL), were significantly reduced. The benefits started at 400 units each day and 1,200 units had added benefit.

(The government recommended daily allowance for Vitamin E is a mere 30 units a day. In order to get these amounts from food you would have to drink pints of vegetable oil or eat pounds of peanut butter each day…just to get 30 units of Vitamin E).

De-generative *dis*-ease occurs slowly and over a period of time.

Study #8:

Performed at the University of California on 11,000 people. Supplementing with Vitamin C, cuts the death rate from heart *dis*-ease in half and lengthens the life expectancy up to 6-years.

Study #9:

Published in *The American Journal of Clinical Nutrition*, May of 1999. The Department of Nutrition at Harvard School of Public Health reported a 10-year study of 76,000 women. Those with the highest intake of Essential Fatty Acids (EFA's or *good fats*), reduced their death rate by 55%.

Some other studies I found showed that 1,000 milligrams to 2,000 milligrams (of good fats), reduces the clumping and stickiness of blood cells to the walls of the arteries, preventing heart attacks. Population studies have shown Vitamin C to raise the good cholesterol and lower the bad cholesterol levels and that combining Vitamins E & C work better than either of the two by themselves.

The New England Journal of Medicine reported that people with high homocysteine levels (a byproduct of metabolism), have 30-times the risk of heart *dis*-ease and that supplementing with Folic Acid, one of the B-Complex vitamins, homocysteine levels decreased.*

*Thirty-years ago, Kilmer McCully, MD, discovered that cholesterol and clogged arteries are not the culprits of heart *dis*-ease. But rather the symptoms of heart *dis*-ease. McCully's pioneering 1969 theory that linked homocysteine, a byproduct of metabolism that accumulates in the blood, was not embraced by the medical-community. His ideas were not popular in the schools and hospitals, so his work was suppressed and ignored...*laughed-off*. In fact, McCully was banished from Harvard University and Massachusetts General Hospital and denied a new position for more than two-years because of his research. His observations went head-to-head with the accepted medical theory of the day.

In fact, more recently, the Landmark Studies I & II showed that consistent use of what I refer to as the B.N.B.B.s dramatically lowers the risk, for ***all the major de-generative dis-eases, of our time:***

http://www.landmarkstudy.com/

Supplemental Calcium:

Calcium supplements have been shown to prevent cholesterol from being reabsorbed in the intestine. Certain kinds of alfalfa supplements actually bind with cholesterol and carry it out of the body. Germany's Commission E (like The Food and Drug Administration), approved garlic for its safety and effectiveness for treatment of some heart *dis*-ease.

A well-known and respected professor and Medical Doctor at the University of North Carolina intended to reduce his cholesterol. In 1980 at age 36 he was a following the lactovegetarian model of eating, meaning he included dairy products, in his diet. He took a food-concentrated, Multi-vitamin known to help reduce cholesterol levels by balancing the body chemistry and supplemented with a well-known, Certified-Organic, Non-GMO, Soy Protein drink mix. His cholesterol was 225.

In 1981 at age 37 he became a vegan, meaning he eliminated animal products from his diet. (The bad cholesterol (LDL) in food is from animal products). He was still taking the Multi-vitamin and Certified-Organic, Non-GMO, Soy Protein. His cholesterol dropped to 220. He added back dairy products to his diet since it made such little difference.

In 1984 at age 40 he added seven-grams of fiber to his diet and added eight-capsules daily of supplemental EPA, an oil from the body of certain fish like salmon and mackerel. His cholesterol dropped 45-points to 175.

In 1994 at age 50, he increased his fiber intake by 15-grams, per day, of a multiple source fiber supplement known to work better than some cholesterol lowering medications. He also began to exercise followed by a properly formulated, post-workout recovery drink (Functional-food), which maximizes energy replacement and fat burning. *His cholesterol dropped another 40 points to 135.*

Another doctor's experience with the B.N.B.B.s:

A female medical doctor, heart specialist and pediatrician had a hiatal hernia, had gained 55-pounds, had severe morning sickness, high blood pressure, migraine headaches, skin problems, hair loss, nail problems, chronic fatigue, premature-ventricular fibrillation, of the heart and her EKG test indicated numerous small heart attacks. She applied principles in alignment with those in this book and all these problems corrected themselves.

Personal Trainer:

Sandy, a Certified Aerobics Instructor, was focused on burning excess body fat and getting lean. She was teaching an aerobics-class one day and she began having chest pains. She ended up in the emergency room thinking she was having a heart attack. This is someone whom thought she ate good and exercised regularly. To make a long story short, the lining around her heart was inflamed and the doctors couldn't find a cause (they haven't been taught to recognize malnutrition and its consequences manifesting on the body), so they just put her on anti-inflammatory drugs, addressing the outward symptom (inflammation), not the cause.

Or in other words, covering up the warning-light with a piece of really expensive and toxic tape. She took the prescription, the inflammation went away and when she ran out of the drug the inflammation came back. Back to the doctor and back on the drugs. Her doctor warned her about the side-effects of the drugs on her kidneys and liver, but he didn't know what else to do since the pain and inflammation were recurrent. An acquaintance at the gym told her about someone else whom the same thing happened to them. They took the good-fats and the problem went away. Sandy began taking a lot of good-fats and to her doctor's dismay the pain and inflammation went away.

Within a couple-months the problem returned again! Sandy realized she ran out of her supplemental good-fats, a couple of months back. Now she takes the good-fats every day whether she thinks she needs them or not and the problem with her heart hasn't returned. *It makes good sense to prevent dis-ease, does it not?*

Nutritional-deficiency shows up differently in every person:

People with un-diagnosable or un-recognizable health problems can feel better by applying these principles.

How do we know heart *dis*-ease occurs over time?

In addition to the increase of *de*-generative *dis*-eases like diabetes and obesity among young people, here are a couple of examples.

One study done reflected the results of autopsies done on 800-children killed in car accidents, whom already showed the signs of heart *dis*-ease developing. Specifically, atherosclerosis or thickening of the walls of the arteries, which leads to blocked arteries and finally heart attack.

Another similar study reflected the results of autopsies performed on young soldiers killed in combat. With an average age of 22-years, the soldiers showed the signs of heart *dis*-ease already developing.

Why such a focus on heart *dis*-ease?

I didn't want to go into a lengthy discussion of every *de*-generative *dis*-ease. There's an easier way. Heart *dis*-ease is the number-one killer in America. Behind the lifestyle habits, which create a lot of heart *dis*-ease, follows all the other *de*-generative *dis*-eases, which nobody wants anyway…I saw no point going into all of them. Up until now, I have focused primarily on the problems with eating fast-energy and junk foods and beverages combined with an absence of the B.N.B.B.s which help prevent all those *de*-generative *dis*-eases.

The circulatory system, endocrine system, reproductive system, respiratory system, muscular system, skeletal system and nervous systems **all require the same nutritional components to maintain themselves**, prevent *dis*-ease and repair themselves…*guess which ones*…the B.N.B.B.s!

So you see, it doesn't make sense to approach the body in a "Black-Forest" of chasing symptoms manner/chasing symptoms with individual-nutrients…*doing so assumes we know exactly which components are needed throughout the body and the chain of events of any given dis-ease breaking down process…but we don't know all the nutritional-components*…only the ones that have already been recognized and named by scientists…so it's sensible to put ***all*** the nutritional components, in the body (B.N.B.B.s) and let nature do the work…*simply provide them.* 'Picking and choosing' interferes with nature picking and choosing, which nutrients your body actually needs…*short-changing Mother Nature's ability to keep you healthier,* regardless of your situation.

Reason 55. Considering or have already had bariatric-surgery?

Bariatric-surgery is when modifications have been made to the digestive system to force people to lose weight, either by limiting how much food can be eaten at a time or by removing a part of the digestive system completely. The upside is that people whom haven't done the necessary exercise and nutritional-modifications, to get healthy, lose 'weight' anyway, regardless the underlying health [symptoms] of their lifestyle habits.

One of the key concepts here is that even in people whom are considered healthy might not be absorbing enough nutrition for long-term prevention of the so common, major *de*-generative *dis-eases*, especially so leading up to AND following bariatric surgery. Even people whom are generally over-weight are considered under-fed, in that even though they are fat, they don't have enough nutrition-density in their body to use the fat for energy and reverse insulin-resistance processes.

The only way to know is whether the patient is having signs, symptoms and clinically measurable deficiencies of the blood chemistry, *e.g. high blood pressure, high cholesterol, high blood sugar, etc.* For a lot of nutrients, there are few accurate tests to measure nutrients levels in the blood.

The people whom have bariatric-surgery have effectively reduced the surface area responsible for the absorption of the very nutrients that would have made it possible to lose fat safely in a healthy manner in the first place!…after surgery, the needed amount of B.N.B.B.s is *increased* equal to the amount of surface area within the digestive system itself, but nutritional-absorption is dramatically decreased!..*thereby increasing the need for supplemental B.N.B.B.s their doctors suggest after the weight loss surgery itself.*

Reason 56. Want beautiful, healthy skin, hair & nails?

Healthy hair, skin and nails starts from the inside out. The hair, skin and nails are literally made out of the B.N.B.B.s, but neither of them stores the nutrition they need in themselves and if that weren't enough, skin, hair and nails get last-call. The quality of your hair, skin and nails is reflective of what's going on in the rest of your body. If yours aren't what you want them to be you need supplemental B.N.B.B.s.

Fitness Magazine published an article entitled, *The 5 Best Vitamins for Hair Growth.*

"Nutrients like Zinc and B-Complex enhance your hair health," summarized Melissa Piliang, MD, a dermatologist at the Cleveland Clinic. The best part?

Vitamin D:

We all know the 'sunshine-vitamin' gives us a much-needed energy boost, but Vitamin D may also stimulates the hair follicle and activates cells within the hair shaft (translation: Grow, baby, grow!). It also helps control your body's mineral balance, specifically Zinc levels, and if it goes off-kilter, symptoms like a flaky scalp and thinning, lackluster hair may start to appear.

Vitamin A:

A true all-around winner, Vitamin A is great for promoting a healthy, moisturized scalp, preventing hair from drying out, keeping dandruff at bay, and regulating retinoic acid (too much of which can lead to hair loss) in the hair follicles...Vitamin A is a powerful antioxidant that we can't do without.

"Basically, every cell of the body needs Vitamin A to function," says dermatologist Cybele Fishman, MD.

"It also helps protect and produce the oils that sustain your scalp, and being low on Vitamin A can even leave you with itchy, irksome dandruff," recommends Greg Hottinger, RD, nutritionist and author of *The Best Natural Foods on the Market Today.*

Vitamin C:

While we've heard countless times that Vitamin C is essential for maintaining a healthy immune system, it can also do wonders for hair growth. It helps build collagen, which stimulates the follicle to lengthen, and helps break down Iron, an essential component of long and strong hair.

"The major reason we need it is that it helps to transport oxygen throughout the body," says Paul Thomas, RD, a scientific consultant to the National Institute of Health.

By facilitating the breakdown of Iron, Vitamin C ensures that the body gets enough oxygen to each cell that works at maintaining healthy hair, skin, and nails.

Vitamin E:

Stimulating the expansion of the capillaries and promoting a strong blood supply is what Vitamin E does best. This means that it helps foster a healthy scalp, which lays the foundation for long, supple hair.

Vitamin H:

Often known by its more common name, Biotin, this vitamin is included in the B-Complex group with other vitamins like Niacin and Cobalamin. (Vitamin H is also called Vitamin B7 and Co-enzyme R). Since research has linked Biotin deficiency to alopecia, or hair loss, it's considered an important vitamin to help strengthen hair and nails.

Reason 57. Senior?:

Tufts University made the nutritional supplements part of the daily food guide pyramid for senior citizens, for a number of reasons, including decreased absorption related to age and decreased numbers of meals consumed by seniors.

Reason 58. Not eating enough fiber?

If you aren't eating 25-50 grams of fiber each day and you really don't know which Whole-foods to eat that are high in fiber, you'll need to take a fiber supplement to get your fiber intake up until you learn enough about Whole-food to get it from food itself.

A study done by one of the most well-respected and renowned nutrition research companies demonstrated that the simple act of eating 15-grams, of fiber per day, (a very little bit) increases the rate at which stuff passes through the body by 45%. That means instead of being a swamp, the body becomes a fast-flowing stream, able to keep itself clean from the inside-out.

There was an article in the September 1987 *Journal of the American Dietetic Association* entitled, *Fiber and Colon Cancer* the authors summarized 40-different studies. Dr. Peter Greewald of the National Cancer Institute concluded that..."*...the association between high fiber intake and lower risk of cancer is consistent, coherent and strong.*"

Reason 59. Eat sugar or high-fructose corn syrup?

These things found in many food and beverage products deplete the body of the B.N.B.B.s, in the sense that they require the B.N.B.B.s, in order for the body to derive energy, assimilate and eliminate the waste of them from the body. Without the B.N.B.B.s, the potential energy of these ingredients get stored, unable to be liberated as energy as well as take the B.N.B.B.s away from all the other systems of the body which should be a higher priority (insulin-resistance). They take away from the body the very nutrients required to process them properly.

For those of you whom know about mining, strip-mining is a good analogy of what these ingredients do to the body: *strip away the natural resources, while leaving a devasted landscape locally and systemically.*

Reason 60. Ever experience stress?

Stress on the body is like driving your automobile hard and fast...it uses up fuel and resources faster and leaves the engine vulnaerable to the effects of use...more likely to *de*-generate.

American Medical Association (AMA) Reports: The following are excerpts from A Seattle Newspaper, Wednesday, June 19, 2002 entitled, *"Take multivitamins, AMA urges:* Journal reverses policy as more benefits surface."

Chicago – "Reversing a long-standing anti-vitamin policy, *The Journal of The American Medical Association* today is advising all adults to take *at least* one Multi-vitamin pill, *each day.*"

"Scientists' understanding of the benefits of vitamins have rapidly advanced, and it now appears that people whom get enough vitamins may be able to prevent such common chronic diseases as cancer, heart dis-ease and osteoporosis," according to Drs. Robert Fletcher and Kathleen Fairfield, of Harvard University, whom wrote the new guidelines.

The last time the *Journal of The American Medical Association (JAMA)* made a comprehensive review of vitamins, about 20-years ago, it concluded people of normal health should not take Multi-vitamins because they were, *"... a waste of time and money." "People can get all the nutrients they need from their diet,"* JAMA advised, adding that, *"...pregnant women and chronically sick people may need certain vitamins."*

Researchers hope *JAMA's* endorsement will encourage more people to reap the health benefits of a daily Multi-vitamin.

Almost 80% of Americans don't eat at least five-helpings of fruits and vegetables a day, the recommended minimum amount believed to provide sufficient essential-nutrients. ***Humans do not make their own vitamins, except for some Vitamin D if they get adequate sunshine, and they must get them from an outside-source to prevent metabolic dis-orders.***

Dr. Jeffrey Blumberg, chief of antioxidant research at Tuft's University's Jean Mayer USDA Human Nutrition Research Center on Aging said, *"...the JAMA recommendations underscore a growing concern among nutrition experts that the recommended daily allowances, or RDAs, for many vitamins are set too low."*

"RDAs essentially were established to prevent symptoms of vitamin-deficiency disorders," he said. ***"But evidence is growing that higher levels of many vitamins are necessary to achieve optimum health,"*** said Dr. Blumberg.

"Even people whom eat five-daily servings of fruits and vegetables may not get enough of certain vitamins for optimum health," Fletcher said. ***"Most people for instance cannot get the healthiest levels of Folate and Vitamins D and E from recommended diets,"*** he said.

"All of us grew up believing that if we ate a reasonable diet, that would take care of our vitamin needs," Fletcher said. ***"But the new evidence, much of it in the last couple-of-years, is that vitamins also prevent the usual diseases we deal with every day- heart disease, cancer, osteoporosis and birth defects."***

"Because foods contain thousands-of-vitamin-like-compounds [many not yet identified] that may be important for good health, vitamin supplements should not be a substitute for a wholesome-diet," Blumberg said. (The three-parts of a complete nutrition program are Whole-foods, Functional-foods and the B.N.B.B.s).

In other studies…

"Most people do not consume an optimal amount of all vitamins by diet alone," write researchers Kathleen M. Fairfield, MD, and Robert H. Fletcher in companion JAMA studies.

Most at risk are elderly, vegans, alcohol consumers and those whom absorb less nutrition than they need.

Moira Lawler wrote an article entitled, *The Vitamin Deficiency That's Hurting Your Workout:*

"It's time to start meeting the daily recommendations for this vitamin."

Deficient in Vitamin D? It could be keeping you from maxing out your athletic prowess. A recent study set to be published in the *International Journal of Sport Nutrition and Exercise Metabolism* found low levels of the vitamin messes with the way your muscles function.

For the study, Oklahoma researchers looked at about 100 college athletes and tracked their Vitamin D and Calcium intake and the amount of time spent in the sun. **Even though the athletes lived in the South, where sunshine is plentiful, many weren't meeting the daily Vitamin D recommendations.** Nearly 1/4 of the athletes logged insufficient levels, which were between 50-and-75 nanomoles per liter (nmol/L). 9% had less than 50 nmol/L, qualifying as Vitamin D deficient. For comparison purposes, the World Health Organization and Endocrine Society says, *"...anything over 75 nmol/L is good to go."*

Stress hormones?: **Studies have shown that nutrients included in the B.N.B.B.s can have a 'buffering' effect on the stress hormones, which get released during physical, psychological and emotional-stress. This is a casual way of saying that the nutrients prevent the stress hormones like cortisol and adrenaline from having such detrimental effects, as they would have without adequate-nutrition circulating in the body. Cortisol for example, tends to concentrate in the area of the body where we store emotional or psychological stress (neck, back, gut) or areas that get stress through repetetive injury and physical use without adequate recovery between sessions (knees, low back, neck, tendons, ligaments, etc).** In my experience as a licensed massage practitioner I worked on muscles where people had chronic stress from work and the muscles were so hard and lacking in circulation and oygen that no matter how much pressure I applied they wanted more, to the point that it didn't seem like they could feel the muscle any more and I didn't feel I could apply more pressure, without rupturing the muscle belly. This is a great example where chronic stress hasn't been balanced with time off, recreation, fun, exercise and the three- parts of nutrition: 1) Whole-foods 2) Functional-foods and 3) B.N.B.B.s.

Chapter Nine

Proper hydration in fitness, sports and atheltic-nutrition...

Reason 61. Hydration during athletic training and events:

It's [impossible] to replace minerals, electrolytes, energy and fluid, *with water alone.*

[[Proper hydration during exercise, training and competitive-events requires the use of Functional-foods. **Whole-foods and water alone take too long to work during the event itself, for the athlete to benefit, from what they consumed during the event itself.** Anyone whom says otherwise is providing an example of 'theory-based nutrition': *it sounds good and boosts their ego, but doesn't provide the fuel the working body needs and actually/literally contributes to heat and hydration injuries...***the number-one reason people are forced to drop out of fitness and athletic events is hydration injuries]].**

Explanation:

Our bodies are 60%-to-80% water.

Water itself is essential for:

● Cooling the body,

● Carrying waste out of the body,

● Delivering nutrients throughout the body,

● Flushing out the toxic byproducts of exercise and daily living and

● Building new tissue, *e.g., muscles, organs, bones, tendons, ligaments, immune system, etc.*

More athletic events are lost due to dehydration (shortage of water, minerals & electrolytes and certain kinds of carbohydrates) than any other cause.

People often *assume they'll know*, when they need more fluids, by their level of thirst. *Not true.* Thirst lags behind need for fluid by about 1.5-to-2 liters.

In other words, by the time you are thirsty you are already dehydrated by 1.5-to-2 liters of fluid.

Being dehydrated means your body is using more fluid than you are drinking and is getting distributed throughout your body, for all the processes associated with training and competition. Cooling the body being one of the primary processes. As you probably know, during a fever, the body gets too hot and a person's ability to function decreases significantly.

(Fluids, electrolytes and certain kinds of carbohydrate make up the bulk of what your focus will be and what you can control in your environment to achieve and exceed your peak performances).

Fluid refers to water and things mixed into water to get it into your system the fastest way, without actually hooking up and IV bag to a blood vein (Functional-foods).

Electrolytes refers to the nutritional-components, in water, which make water work better. These will be covered in detail shortly.

Energy refers to food-type things we ingest in order to have energy to function and in this context, it also refers to [putting energy back into the body] before, during and after training and competitions (specifically, carbohydrates).

During daily life, exercise, training and competition, the body cools itself three ways:

1. ● Exhaling,

2. ● Exposure to air cooler than the body and

3. ● Sweating - When we produce more heat than the body can cool the first two ways, we sweat.

Sweat consists of [fluids] taken, *from within the body* and [electrolytes] taken, *from within the body.* Both of which, are from what we put into our body. Sweat is secreted onto the skin to cool the body. It also balances the acid-level, of the body, which rises during exercise, training and competition. An effect of acidity is pain and fatigue of the muscles.

1) The chemical reactions that make it possible to train at higher levels slow down. For example, water must be available in adequate amounts in order for your body to convert stored carbohydrates into energy usable for the brain, heart and muscles to function.

When you do not have enough water in your body...

2) Cells cannot function to maintain, repair or rebuild tissues effectively. Meaning a person whom drinks too little water on a consistent basis, will be injury prone, recover slowly from workouts, feel sluggish and heavy, less alert and the immune system will function at a slower rate...*lacking the edge.*

3) Toxins build up in the body, making peak performance impossible.

4) Stones in the kidneys and bladder are more likely. *The Journal of Sports and Fitness* published an article stating that marathon competitors have six-times the risk of kidney stones, as a result of inadequate hydration.

Your level of hydration is reflected in the way you look, feel, think and perform.

Even mild dehydration can lower performance levels of exercise, mental alertness, learning and memory, recovery from illness, prevention of *dis*-ease and immune function as well as the quality of your skin, hair, nails, eyes and lips.

Just for the fun of it...

A 150-pound person has about 11-gallons of water in their body. One gallon of water weighs 8-pounds. (11 x 8 = 88 pounds).

A person whom hardly does anything uses up about ¾ of a gallon, each day.

A person sitting in the desert uses up about 2½-gallons-a-day, the same used during a marathon. That's about 8%-to-9% of total body weight.

In many athletic events, if the competitor drops just 5% of their body weight during competition, they are disqualified...*that's how important water is*. According to Liz Vaccariello, editor of the magazine *Fitness*, 75% of Americans are chronically dehydrated resulting in fatigue, increased blood pressure and headaches.

The American Medical Athletic Association says, *"...an average of 318 Americans die, each year, from heat-related illness, brought on by dehydration. Many, many more suffer from it. You don't have to be one of them. It's one of those sports-related illnesses that is preventable."*

The drink of choice, according to Dr. Noel Nequin, of the American Medical Athletic Association is a quality sports drink. Research shows that a lightly-flavored sports drink encourages people to drink up to 90% more than just plain water. And that's a good thing because kids are at greater risk from heat illness than adults. Their smaller bodies produce more heat and sweat less than adults, all of which limit their ability to cool themselves. The more your kids hydrate while they are outside, enjoying sports, nature and all the good things that happen to kids in motion, the better they will feel.

Results of fluid loss on peak performance…

0% loss:

- Peak performance

2% loss:

- Feel weaker

4% loss:

- Breathing harder

5% loss:

- Muscles won't go

6% - 8% loss:

- Dizzy,

- Really fatigued,

- Disorientation,

- Increased heart rate,

- Increased respiration,

- Decreased coordination.

- Limbs feel like they have weights attached.

- You will rest!! No matter how hard you try, you're going to be on the ground!

In order to determine how much water you use up, weigh yourself before and after your training sessions and competitions, without clothing or gear. Take serious note of how much weight-loss you experience.

If your before-and-after weight difference is…

2% or more of your bodyweight, your performance suffered.

3%-to-4% of your bodyweight, there are potential risks, including elevated heart rate and increased body temperature.

Prevent this from happening by consuming more fluids, before and during training and events.

Then, drink 16-ounces of fluid, for every pound of body weight you lost, during training/events in the form of a [complete] sports drinks and [properly formulated] muscle recovery drink, within the first couple-of-hours after training/event. Then, when you feel full of those, continue with water until your body weight is restored prior to training again (within 24-hours).

As a side note: contrary to myth, weighing yourself on a scale is not a reliable way to calculate a decrease in body fat. If you weigh less after your workouts, it means you have lost water that must be replaced before you train, exercise or compete again or else your performance will not be what it could and you could potentially require emergency medical care.

Electro-what's?.. so, what?

In order for the body to functional optimally, electrolyte-levels must remain nearly constant, along with water. If electrolyte-levels decrease, within the body, they must be replaced (before the next workout) or performance drops off. Electrolytes have to be in the body in order for water to get into and out of the cells of the body. Sweating, bleeding, breathing, using the restroom, diarrhea, fever, vomiting, burns and wounds cause the loss of electrolytes. Electrolytes are so important that as you have probably seen on television or through your own experience, IV bags are one of the first things done for people whom are sick or injured, because they bring the body back into balance. *IV bags contain water and electrolytes and sometimes glucose.*

Without water, *minerals and electrolytes cannot do their job.*

Without minerals and electrolytes, water cannot do its job efficiently.

In other words, water follows electrolytes into and throughout the cells of the body. ***Without the proper amounts/ratios of electrolytes, water cannot get into or out of the cells.*** The body becomes stagnant like a swamp and it's reflected in performance. Other than keeping the body cool and detoxifying the body, water is essential because without water, carbohydrates cannot be stored or released for energy. Specific ratios of the electrolytes have to be present in a sports drink, otherwise the drink is just a sugary, salty drink….which won't get you close to your top performances.

The key electrolytes and their benefits to you:

Now, before I go over the absolutely necessary electrolytes a [complete sports drink] must contain, here is another question for you and your team mates and training partners. As you look over the benefits of each electrolyte in the list below, imagine yourself working out, training or competing...

"Which of these benefits are you willing to skip or go without?"

By purposely with-holding the B.N.B.B.s and/or Functional-foods, this is exactly what you're doing.

Sodium:

• Maintains fluid balance, preventing dehydration.

• Maintains acid balance, delaying onset of fatigue.

• Nerve transmission, makes it possible for your muscles to keep working, delaying fatigue.

• Helps maintain proper body temperature, preventing overheating.

• Keeps heart working optimally.

Potassium:

- Helps convert carbohydrates to usable energy.

- Helps convert protein to amino acids for maintenance and repair of muscle.

- Nerve-transmission, makes it possible for your muscles to keep working.

- Keeps heart working optimally.

- Prevents cramps.

- Allows tolerance to heat.

- Proper reflexes.

- Mental alertness.

- Muscular strength and endurance

Calcium:

- Muscle contractions.

- Nerve-transmission, makes it impossible for your muscles to keep working.

- Strong, damage resistant, faster healing bones.

Phosphorus:

- Energy transfer of cells, making stored energy available for use by muscles.

- Maintains acid balance, delaying onset of fatigue.

Chloride:

• Maintains acid balance, delaying onset of fatigue.

• Maintains fluid volume, preventing cramps, overheating and loss of strength.

• Regulates potassium loss…*all of potassium benefits.*

Magnesium:

• Helps turn carbohydrates into energy usable by muscles.

• Helps make protein available to muscles for repair and maintenance.

• Muscle relaxation, preventing cramping.

• 300 different chemical reactions involving muscle strength and clear thinking.

Going without any one of them will decrease your performance significantly. Does it make sense to use a [complete] sports drink or just grab random, sweetened, colored-water off the shelf that implies better performance, but doesn't deliver?

Are you willing to give up energy, from the carbohydrates you eat?

Are you willing to give up being able to optimally contract or relax your muscles?

Are you willing to decrease your body's ability to repair muscles after working out?

Are you willing to increase the acid levels within your body during training?

Do you want your heart to beat regularly without skipping beats?

Do you want to overheat and have to drop out of competition?

Sounds kind of ridiculous, doesn't it? That's exactly what we are doing when we do not (proactively) replace these things during and after athletic activity. It's exactly what you risk when you eat junk and fast-energy foods and beverages.

Drink, drink, drink.

If the fluid level drops in the body, from either sweating or any of the other reasons listed above, less blood flows to and from the heart and lungs, making the heart work harder and faster to get oxygen and nutrient rich blood to muscles, leaving the body feeling fatigued, unable to come even close to optimal performance.

Most people, athletes and non-athletes, induce voluntary dehydration simply because they think they aren't thirsty even when there are drinks around them to consume. **Thirst should [not] be considered an adequate indicator of need by the body for fluid.**

Thirst is not sensed until a person is dehydrated by 1.5-to-2 liters of fluid. By that time, there is no way to catch up to a properly hydrated state during training or competition…the body simply cannot make up the difference, fast enough, if fluid consumption started at the same time the thirst sensation was noticed!

Water vs a sports drink:

Refueling the body is not as simple as eating food or drinking a sugary drink. For the most part, the digestive system shuts down during exercise. Water by itself is absorbed too slowly to do any good during the training session or event. The people, professionals and non-professionals alike, whom say differently simply don't know any better…*yet.*

Now, go have a new personal best!

A clinical study on trained athletes:

A group of experienced runners was divided into three smaller groups and told to, *"Run until they couldn't."* They were running at 85% of their VO2 max or in other words, 85% of their maximum ability.

• Group one drank nothing and lasted 54-minutes.

• Group two drank water alone and lasted 78-minutes.

• Group three drank a fluid, electrolyte, energy mixture like the one I describe and ran 122-minutes.

Effective hydration and energy:

In this next example, highly trained cyclists rode stationary cycles for 200-minutes at 45% of their maximum ability. Group one was given flavored water (the equivalent of an incomplete sports drink) and rode at 85% of their maximum. They were able to ride for an additional 2-minutes.

Group two was given a combination drink designed to replenish fluids (water), energy (carbohydrates), and the 6-key minerals and electrolytes and also instructed to ride at 85% of their max. This group was able to ride 31-minutes longer than the flavored water group.

Consistency:

In order to consistently perform and feel your best…and for that matter...improve your performance by 20%, drink about 25-grams of a combination of carbohydrates: a combination of glucose (very fast-energy), fructose (fast and long lasting), and maltodextrin (slower, but longer-lasting along with 100-grams of sodium per ½ hour of activity. Calcium, Magnesium, Potassium, Chloride and Phosphorus will dramatically boost performance. I mean *really boost performance.*

And this combination goes right into your bloodstream for instant use, without the delay of digestion

The American College of Sports Medicine recommends drinking your sports drink about 15-minutes before your event.

Food and beverage taste differently and are tolerated differently by the body during activity and non-active times. Cool and slightly sweetened is appetizing, "*...regardless of whether the activity lasts a half-hour or longer than four-hours, there is no question that athletes should get in the habit of drinking a sports beverage, rather than water. Consumption of sports beverages results in better performance than water whether you do sprints or endurance work,*" says Dan Bernardot, Ph.D, RD.

Other factors that can change these general guidelines:

• Humidity level,

• Temperature of air,

• Intensity of training,

• Your personal fitness level and

• Your body's idiosyncrasies.

If you and/or your team mates have been drinking only water, or [incomplete sport drinks] before (meaning drinks that don't contain the above ingredients or contain other unnecessary filler ingredients), during and after training and competition you haven't experienced peak performance...*yet*...you're missing out.

If the teams you are competing against have been drinking only water, I would have to say you all have been moving in slow motion compared to what you'll experience by applying these principles. Ask me for help.

Sweating, breathing, using the bathroom and exercising all cause the body to use up water.

"Water is all you need"…wrong.

I often hear so-called experts say water is all that is needed to replace the water-level, within the body and that sport drinks are, *"a waste of money"… this isn't true, but* **some are** *a waste of energy.* [That is both true and false]. A lot of sport drinks *are* a waste of money because they are marketed as complete sports drinks, but lack all/some of the six-minerals and electrolytes, mentioned above and go so far as to add in ingredients that don't have any place in performance nutrition and in some cases add ingredients that aren't healthy, and even inhibit optimal functioning of the body, under intense training and competitive environments.

If you could add a [precise amount of sodium] to the water, it would get absorbed almost as quickly as you drink it.

Add glucose polymers (fast-acting sugars that provide long-term energy), and the water gets absorbed even faster than with the salt alone.

You do need water, but (during training and events) water is absorbed too slowly to do any good for athletes both training and in competition. As I said earlier, water follows electrolytes. *Without the proper mixture of electrolytes, water just sits in the gut* for a long time before being absorbed. All the while, the body is still using up water (faster than it's being absorbed). In other words, your body is using up the water faster than it's being replaced.

During intense physical exertion, the digestive system shuts down to a degree as blood is distributed to the muscles. That's why it usually doesn't make any sense to eat a lot of solid food before or during training and competition (except during ultra-long events). Much of the digestive process shuts down because the blood is going to the muscles.

By adding the glucose polymers to the water, energy can be replaced as fast as it is being used up. Not only to raise the instant energy level (blood sugar), but also to store energy in the muscles and liver for later use. Isn't that awesome!

Amount is critical:

Another reason effective sport drinks work so well is that they are premixed to match the chemistry of the body, the same way IV fluids are (IV fluids aren't random mixtures). So, the body doesn't have to do any work in order to utilize the minerals, electrolytes and glucose polymers.

If you have ever drunk a really sweet drink and shortly after began experiencing stomach cramps and diarrhea, that's exactly what I'm talking about, in terms of poor quality or a poorly-formulated/ineffective sport drink. This also happens with fruit juice that is too concentrated (too much sugar at one time).

If the sugar level is too high or too concentrated, the body has to bring water from other areas of the body in order to "water it down" so it can be used, for energy. But often, because of the "more is better" way of thinking, the level of sugar (and salt) is so high that the body just dumps the fluid into the large intestine, where suddenly the consumer feels as if they have to go to the bathroom. Along with dumping the sugar and water, electrolytes get dumped too and the consumer is left feeling a little shaky and weak. Definitely not what you want any time around training and competition. *I know from experience.*

In general, when using a quality/effective sport drink, the more you consume (of the correct formula), the faster it's absorbed, by the digestive system. The colder the drink, the faster absorption occurs.

So, too much sugar (too concentrated) = diarrhea and slow or no passage of fluid to bloodstream + water is taken away from the muscles that need it.

Too little sugar (too dilute) = not enough energy to replace energy at the speed activity is using it up.

Exceptions to this are digestive problems, the formulation of the drink and how conditioned you are. In other words, by applying these principles consistently you'll be able to train your body to take in higher amounts of this perfect formulation. Start small and slow and build up over time. Begin applying these principles before your events so you can get used to the effects and to calibrate how your body responds. Competition is not the time for experimentation.

The do and the do-nots:

Can you imagine the difference between the athletes whom utilize this practice during competition and the ones whom do not?

The difference is like night and day.

The athletes whom do not will look and feel as if they are moving in slow motion, *compared to you.*

Those of you whom do apply these principles:

Will experience an energy level that stays at a consistently high level, *throughout the competition,* beginning to end. Your mental alertness will be consistent and your muscles will be working at peak capacity, without the effects of lactic acid and fatigue, right through to the end of competition.

And after competition, the usual soreness, cramping and fatigue will be greatly reduced to say the least, by utilizing these principles and after training and competition from, applying the muscle recovery principles. Energy storage and recovery will be faster and dramatically greater than those whom do not apply them. *Now you have the edge!*

Let's review the carbohydrate sources in your sport drink that should be included:

20-to-28 grams per 8-ounces, of fluid, of the following combination is ideal:

Glucose polymers like maltodextrin (unrefined sugar from food) = moves faster than water. Speeds absorption (into the cells of the body) and provide greater muscle glycogen (muscle energy), storage than simple sugars and more stable blood sugar.

Some fructose restores muscle and liver energy stores and is 4-times more efficient at restoring liver-carbohydrate storage. Fructose (sugar from fruit/also low-glyemic), loads the liver and keeps it loaded efficiently. So, there are carbohydrates ready to roll at the sprint (end), part of the race or competition, *e.g., last quarter, final heat, last set, last hundred meters, etc.* In other words, when your competition is running on fumes, your body is fully loaded with the fuel needed to perform at your max!

Glucose is a simple, fast-energy sugar that provides instant energy. Glucose is one of the fastest acting sugars in the body. As an athlete, you do not want to wait for your body to digest the sugars in order to be able to get energy from them. This is one place that it is essential to eat simple, fast-acting sugar.

Hint, hint...

[Hopefully, you've read my book *Results! Performance Nutrition Training.* If you did, you understand how important the B.N.B.B.s are. In order for these awesome fuel and energy sources to be utilized, you have to consume enough of the B.N.B.B.s on a day-to-day basis]. Without enough of the B.N.B.B.s, your body will not be able to use the liquid energy you're putting in your body during the events and training sessions.

The vitamins, minerals and other nutritional building blocks have to be present in your body prior to activity.

Without the B.N.B.B.s you'll drink the energy sources and they will not be able to do their job. It's like a race car that's has a full gas tank, but does not have spark plugs to run the engine.

Karen Asp says, *"There's certain supplements every guy needs."*

Despite what you've read in the sports pages, there are still a few pills out there that won't have you testifying before congress, from unwittingly using supplements containing banned substances. Here's your guide to the supplements you should be taking based on Karen's suggestions:

Multi-vitamin/mineral:

No rocket science here, but it's surprising just how many guys still don't take a multi. The key to makin' em work is to make them part of your routine. Instead of stashing the bottle on a shelf, keep it by your toothbrush or coffee pot—something you hit every day without fail. Make sure your multi also contains two-key nutrients: Selenium (for its cancer protective effects) and Zinc (which helps you make sperm and is largely responsible for the immune system's health). Also, check the capsule size and dosage.

Fish Oil:

Fish is one of the best sources of Omega-3 fatty acids, which are crucial for brain and heart health and act as a natural anti-inflammatory—especially beneficial if you have sports injuries or aching joints. Even if you manage to eat the two-to-three recommended servings of fish each week, Carlson still suggests popping one-to-three grams of fish oil daily, veering toward the higher side if fish isn't really your meat of choice. Also, look for a brand that contains both EPA and DPA, the two key healthy-fats in fish. Get the kind of EPA/DHA supplements, that are from fish harvested in the cold, Northern, less-polluted waters.

Pro-biotics:

These are good bacteria—the same kind found in your intestine—that aid with overall gut health and enhance your immune system. You can get *pro*-biotics in your diet by eating yogurt, fermented and unfermented milk, miso, tempeh, and some juices and soy beverages. However, if you're not eating those foods regularly, take a *pro*-biotic supplement with at least 10-billion live bacteria, from one or more of the Lactobacillus family. It's generally best to take one capsule before bed.

If you're in your 30s, add these to the base plan:

Vitamin D:

Along with boosting bone health, Vitamin D may help prevent diabetes, metabolic syndrome, multiple sclerosis, certain cancers, and other health conditions. Yet, if you're not drinking milk or getting small doses of unprotected sun exposure (your skin makes Vitamin D from sunlight), you could be D-deficient. Surveys have actually found that about 40%-to-70% of children are already deficient, which is why Anding calls this, *"...the new epidemic"*. Recommended allowances call for 400 IU daily, although Anding says, *"... this may be too low"*. Kidney patients may need more.

Glucosamine and Chondroitin:

"These substances, which are found naturally in the body, could be a natural way to help with pain from sports injuries or aching joints," Susan Carlson, Ph.D says, *"Take 1,500 milligrams daily; you should see improvements in six-weeks. If not, those particular ones are probably not working for you"*.

Co-enzyme Q10:

This little gem provides energy for the heart and helps produce ATP, the major energy source for cells. It's also crucial if you're on cholesterol-lowering medications called statins. *"Statins can significantly slow or reduce Co-enzyme Q10, which your heart needs,"* Dr. Jonny Bowden, Ph.D, says. *"Even if you're not on statins, you could give your heart a healthy boost by taking 30-to-60-grams, per day. Otherwise, if you're taking statins, the dose may be higher, perhaps 10- milligrams or more; talk with your physician if you want, although Bowden warns that many physicians aren't well-versed in nutrition"*. I take 200mg – 400 mg per day.

Combined with a Multi-vitamin/mineral, Zinc and Vitamin-E Complex, this combination is referred to as the, *"...natural form of Viagra™"*.

Chapter Ten

The soup

Reason 62. The Soup:

The basic level of the body, organized just above the DNA/RNA level, is the chemistry of the body. A complex 'soup' of chemicals that control and communicate with each other, throughout the brain-body. Without the B.N.B.B.s, not only are the full-development of the body chemicals limited, the chemicals themselves are limited in what they can do on their own and in partnership, *with all the other system and capabilities of the brain-body.*

Dr. Nancy Snyderman, MD, of NBC's Today Show says, *"How well you feed yourself and how hydrated you are,"* means the difference between getting a migraine or not. *"The life you live has a huge impact on whether you get a migraine...take charge of your health,"* says Snyderman.

Reason 62. Relationships?

The brain that does not have enough B.N.B.B.s will not be able to get along well with others.

The qualities needed to get along with others, *e.g. forethought, empathy, compassion, learning-from-mistakes, maturity, impulse-control, good-judgment, conscience, attention, recognizing love and affection and so forth,* depend on the upper-brain (pre-frontal cortex), to be adequately *nutritionally-fueled and nourished.*

A person whom doesn't get enough B.N.B.B.s will have a difficult time getting along with others and repairing relationships that aren't what they want them to be.

In the 1980's *Perspective* Magazine reported that marriage counselor Mary Jane Hungerford, a family counselor for 10-years, said, *"Nutrition is involved in 90% of my cases and in 75% of them, it is a major factor."*

Her claims are supported by an official at the Brunswick Psychiatric Hospital in Amityville, New York, whom noted that 50% of their case load over a 20-year period involved nutritional-*dis*-orders.

Dr. H.L. Newbold, *East-West Journal, March 1979,* a New York psychiatrist concludes, *"I have seen people on the verge of a divorce because their nutritional-problems were so severe. But these problems tend to fade away when you get people away from bad foods and onto a good nutritional-plan."*

Daniel Amen, MD, author of *Change Your Mind, Change You Life,* says *"...nutrition is a major factor in the health of the structure AND the ability of the brain to function optimally is dependant on nutritional supplements."* (The B.N.B.B.s).

Amen says, *"When you optimize your brain everything in your life is better."*

Healthychildren.org shared an article for dietary-supplements for children entitled, *Supplementation for Some Children,* in November 2015.

For some children, however, supplementation may be important. Your child may need some vitamin and/or mineral supplementation, if your family's dietary practices limit the food groups available to him/her. For example, if your household is strictly vegetarian, with no eggs or dairy products (which is not a diet recommended for children), she may need supplements of Vitamins B12 and D as well as Riboflavin and Calcium. Rickets, for example, is a *dis*-ease in which the bones soften, and it is associated with inadequate Vitamin D intake and decreased exposure to sunlight; although uncommon in the United States, it continues to be reported especially in children with darker-pigmented skin. Consult your pediatrician about which supplements are needed and the amounts if they have experience getting positive results with B.N.B.B.s. If they don't, feel free to refer them to me.

Iron-deficiency:

Iron-deficiency does occur among some young children and can lead to anemia (a condition that limits the ability of the blood to carry oxygen). In many cases, the problem is dietary. Toddlers need to receive at least 15-milligrams of Iron, per day, in their food, but many fail to do so. Drinking large quantities of milk may lead to Iron-deficiency anemia, as the child will be less interested in other foods, some of which are potential sources of Iron.

Too Much Milk?

If your child is drinking 24-to-32 ounces (720–960 ml), of milk or less each day, there's little cause for concern. If she drinks much more than that and you can't get her to eat more Iron-rich foods, consult your pediatrician about adding an Iron-supplement to her diet. In the meantime, decrease her milk intake and keep offering her a wide variety of Iron-rich foods so that, eventually, supplementation won't be necessary.

Should children take dietary-supplements? By Dr. Andrew Myers

"It's no secret that children can be picky-eaters. But their growth and development are dependent upon nutrition, from birth all the way through their teenage-years. So, it's important to ensure that children are getting a full, balanced range of vital nutrients throughout their early lives and supplementation can help," says Dr. Andrew Myers.

Dr. Meyers says, *"The mainstay of children's nutritional-supplements is the old reliable children's Multi-vitamin. Multi-vitamins are a perfect addition to your child's daily-diet. They provide supportive nutrition that can help meet the needs of fast-growing, highly-active bodies and minds. Make sure your child's multi contains antioxidants like Vitamins C and E to support growth, the Beta-carotene form of Vitamin A for healthy vision, and B-Complex vitamins and minerals, for healthy bone, heart and immune function."*

Research also demonstrates the importance of ensuring that your child gets plenty of Omega-3 fatty acids, specifically DHA. Omega-3 is critical to the development of children's brain and eyes. And while many children don't like fish (which are terrific sources of Omega-3), kid-friendly EPA/DHA supplements are readily available.

Choose a Multi-vitamin/mineral formulated for your child's age group, one that provides enough of the children's the B.N.B.B.s to keep your child healthier and help them feel better.

Keep in mind that a Multi-vitamin/mineral is no substitute for Whole-foods, but makes up 1/3 of the complete nutrition program. And remember that a vitamin doesn't do any good if your child won't take it. Getting your kids to want to take something that's good for them is half-the-battle.

I have complete B.N.B.B. nutrition programs available in forms children love to take.

Children's survey:

A survey published by Regan L. Bailey, Jaime J. Gahche, Paul R. Thomas, & Johanna T. Dwyer talked about the reason children give for why they use supplements:

Why US children use dietary-supplements:

Background:

Dietary-supplements are used by 1/3 of children. We examined motivations for supplement use in children, the types of products used by motivations, and the role of physicians and health care practitioners in guiding choices about supplements.

Methods:

We examined motivations for dietary-supplement use reported for children (from birth-to-19-years of age; $n = 8,245$)

using the National Health and Nutrition Examination Survey 2007–2010.

Results:

Dietary-supplements were used by 31% of children; many different reasons were given as follows: to 'improve overall health' (41%), to 'maintain health' (37%), for "supplementing the diet" (23%), to 'prevent health problems' (20%), and to 'boost immunity' (14%). Most children (~90%) whom use dietary-supplements use a Multi-vitamin/mineral or Multi-vitamin product. Supplement users tend to be Non-Hispanic white, have higher family incomes, report more physical activity, and have health insurance. Only a small group of supplements used by children (15%) were based on the recommendation of a physician or other health care provider.

Conclusion:

Most supplements used by children are not under the recommendation of a health care provider. The most common reasons for use of supplements in children are for health promotion, yet little scientific data support this notion in nutrient-replete children.

The use of dietary-supplements has increased in the last 30-years in the United States. Parents whom use dietary-supplements are more likely to have children whom use them. Approximately 1/3 of infants, children, and adolescents (from birth-to-19-years of age, henceforth referred to as children) in the United States are reported to use dietary-supplements. However, the actual motivations for use of dietary-supplements among children remain unclear. The purpose of this analysis was to examine motivations for use of dietary-supplements by children, to characterize the types of products that are commonly used, and to update previous estimates of dietary-supplement use among children using the National Health and Nutrition Examination Survey (NHANES), 2007–2010.

In the period 2007–2010, 31% of children reported the use of dietary-supplements in the past month, with no differences by sex. When children less than 2-years of age were excluded, there was a significant inverse trend toward lower dietary-supplement use, with increasing age. Dietary-supplements were more frequently used by Non-Hispanic white children than by Non-Hispanic black or Hispanic children. Children with private health insurance were more likely to report using dietary-supplements than those with public or no health insurance. Weight status, poverty–income ratio, and time spent in front of a computer, television, or video game screen were all inversely related to dietary-supplement use. The vast majority of children took one (86%, SE=1) or two (10%, SE=1) dietary-supplements (data not shown) in the past 30-days.

I can't tell you how many times I have heard people ask, *"If this is true, how come my doctor hasn't told me about it?"*

Chapter Eleven

Reason 63.

"Why hasn't my doctor spoken with me about the B.N.B.B.s...yet"

To me, its so interesting (peculiar, really) that so many agencies and experts tell the public to ask their doctor which supplements to take and for their doctor to determine whether the patient should take supplements [yet, doctors, by their inherent medical school training have the least amount of nutrition training of most any health care providers] (two-hours as an elective if they choose to attend)...best case scenrio, a doctor is going to refer their patient to a Registered Dietician...Registered dieticians are often part of an education system which says we get enough from food when the very surveys they perform show the majority of the population does not get enough nutrition from food...*you tell me.*

I don't know why, here are a few possibilities:

Many doctors want to offer the very best nutritional-advice to their patients, as well as other models of healing, but once the sign an agreement to provide services to Medicaid/Medicare patients they aren't permitted to do so. Even if they have a private practice of their own, on the side, they aren't permitted to offer services like dietary-supplement counseling, to their patients. They can only offer what is covered by the government programs...*isn't that weird?* People are told to consult their doctor for dietary-supplement advice but, in reality, the doctor might not be allowed to provide the information and many dieticians are recommending against the use of dietary-supplements?...*hmmm.* I've met a lot of physicians whom want to offer advice on modalities, like nutritional-supplementation, but can't figure out how to do it without violating the contract they have with their employer or government subsidized health care (Medicaid/Medicare).

Maybe your doctor has not read the clinical studies: There are over 3,000 peer-reviewed medical journals available to health-care providers today; *there is simply no way for every doctor to keep up with all the information!*

Maybe your doctor hasn't experienced benefits herself/himself, yet: There is a major difference between health–care providers whom talk about nutrition with their patients and health-care providers whom take the B.N.B.B.s and apply results-based nutrition, as described herein. If your health-care provider is not taking the B.N.B.B.s everyday they simply will not know what you are missing out on nor will they be able to make accurate nutrition assessments or suggestions. Nor are they likely to believe that the results you are getting are from the improvements to your nutritional program.

After your doctor graduated from medical school he or she may have stopped learning: Many doctors go into medicine for the right reasons but once they become part of the westernized medicine associations they have to choose between getting contracts with health management organizations (HMOs) and learning what they were not provided by the medical school they attended. And if your doctor has not been consistently using the B.N.B.B.s they don't know what a great impact they can have on people's lives. After medical school, physicians choose for the most part what they will study, as it should be.

For the most part, adequate nutrition is not taught in most medical schools: Every medical school in America has its own agenda and its own proprietary teaching methods. In some of the very best medical schools medical students have less than two-hours of nutrition training available to them…and those two-hours are elective, not required. I know of only one medical school which has a program that teaches the information you hold in your hands here. If your physician is not applying the B.N.B.B.s in their own body they simply will not have a clue what their pateints are missing out on.

It's not your doctor's specialty: The Westernized-model of medicine is to make doctors experts in specific areas of the body, *e.g. foot doctor, eye doctor, heart doctor, etc.* Specialists know a lot about an area or system of the body. You see the body is an amazing biological-machine, with many systems which interact and depend on balance of all the other systems. Specialist doctors can be like an arm that is not connected to the body, the arm does not seem to work because it requires all the other systems in order to function. There might be something wrong with the shoulder or back muscles which interfere with the functioning of the arm but the arm specialist only knows about the arm.

And to top it off, HMOs often require the general-practitoners (doctors whom know about *all* the systems of the body), refer their patients to specialists. I cannot tell you how mant times people have told me they went to their "specialist" whom told them everything-about-everything having to do with their health problem but offered no solution other than a drug to cover up the symptoms the body is communicating. Specialsts by nature, know the functions of each system they specialize in, yet often fail to recognize that function is the results of properly nourished cells when energy & information, DNA/RNA, body chemistry, tissues, organs, systems and finally basic structure have as much of the B.N.B.B.s they need.

Your doctor may be under pressure by the hospital, clinic or even the patient, to promote drugs and treatments that insurance will pay for: In many clinics and hospitals the physicians' contract stipulates they must not talk about products, services or treatments which the hospital does not make money on.

Many doctors have not discovered the benefits of 'prevention' yet, and or how to make a living at it; Many doctors are taught in medical school that *dis*-ease is not preventable, just treatable…and we know anything can be successfully treated whether the patient survives the treatment is the question. *"The treatment was a success!..but, the patient did not make it."*

There are a lot of cheap, worthless, good-for-nothing marketing companies, products and scammers out there, it takes time to learn what's what, so it's no wonder your doctor is skeptical: If your doctor is not consistently using the B.N.B.B.s, in concentrated-food-form, they are not likely to even provide moral support in your use of the B.N.B.B.s. There's 85,000 supplements on the market at any given time.

See your doctor if you want your dis-ease 'treated' or the signs and symptoms covered up: Most physicians training is limited to diagnosing *dis*-ease, but then…instead of addressing the real problem, covering up the symptoms, while the real problem state goes unchanged. There are exceptions to this.

Many doctors simply do not have the time to study it: And since they do not "study" it, they have not rationalized applying it. HMOs require doctors see a certain number of patients, every hour (something like one patient, every nine-minutes), in order to fulfill their contract. Many doctors do not know what to suggest nutritionally, so they refer patients to Registered dieticians whom are practicing [theory-based] nutrition, based on outdated nutriton standards, suggesting we can get what we need from food alone (*nutrition information that pre-dates the state of the soil in the 1930's!*).

Your doctor's liability insurance may not cover giving advice about non-prescription medical modalities.

*Your doctor's peers may belittle nutrition and consider it secondary to 'real' medicine…*you know, the kind that does not teach medical students that the body is made up of the B.N.B.B.s.

It's really up to you to take responsibilty and prevent the degenerative dis-ease process: If you wait until your doctor tells you to take the B.N.B.B.s everyday, you may suffer or even die before the American Medical Associations admits how important *all* the B.N.B.B.s are. And if you are following the guidelines, within this book, you are safe since we only use concentrated food-form B.N.B.B.s. Your doctor simply cannot provide the kind of time and energy you need because there are hundreds-of-other-patients, to take care of and the top ten *dis*-eases (obesity, diabetes, heart *dis*-

ease, cancer, etc.), are largely related to lifestyle factors anyway, e.g. …(the things you do as part of your daily routine, e.g. *what you eat, how well you exercise, what you think about and whether you consume the B.N.B.B.s or not).*

If you do not take care of yourself there is nothing your doctor can do, but watch you de-generate: Many people are ruining their health with their lifestyle choices and then go to their doctor to get something to cover up the signs that the body needs better nutrition.

Some doctors would rather treat the dis-ease than help you build health: Most doctors simply teach what they were taught in medical school and often the medical school has to teach what the pharmaceutical company that sponsored the school wants to be taught…in other words, if drugs to cover up the symptoms of too few B.N.B.B.s are not taught and carried out in practice, the money to the school is cut off. Medical school students usually do not know what they will be taught or what the agenda of their particular school is until they are way into their medical education.

Some doctors think their patients just want a pill to cover up the symptom: See your doctor for annual checkups, emergencies and necessary, unavoidable surgeries. Take optimal care of yourself with the B.N.B.B.s. If you do not take care of yourself there is nothing your doctor can do but watch you *de*-generate. A large percentage of patients whom go to the E.R. only want treatments that their insurance will cover, even if it's a widely available, low-cost OTC medication.

In many cases patients demand the drugs even though the doctors think there are better alternatives: Doctors know that all drugs are toxic and have side-effects, which promote *de*-generative *dis*-ease.

Some physicians hate to have their judgement questioned, especially by people they consider lay-people: In some cases the very ego that drives physicians through medical school is the very ego that prohibites physicians from really hearing what you say or from considering options they were not taught about in medical school. If your physician has such an underdeveloped personality that they will not give you moral support that you might think you need at first, get other people to support you….maybe get a second opinion…or a third…or a fourth.

Sometimes doctors miss things: Doctors spend their entire professional lives learning new information and about 1/2 of what was considered valid, at the time, changes every ten-years. Medical schools teach that in ten-years, what the medical students learn today, 50% will be invalid.

The following is an excerpt from Dr. Atkins book, *Vita-Nutrient Solution* pages 368-369:

To begin with, the establishment oganizations feel that *"The best nutritional-strategy, for optimal health, is to obtain adequate-nutrients, from a wide variety of foods. Supplementation is not appropriate unless scientific evidence of safety and effectiveness is well-accepted."*

In other words, they continue to reject all the scientific-evidence I have shown you, in which vita-nutrients have proven effective dosages, beyond those in normal diet.

Knowing that the insider groups have all endorsed the same positions allows them to fall back on the term 'scientific agreement', which they recognize as the basis for the recommended daily allowances and which they insist should serve as the maximum dosage, should a person wish to take supplemental B.N.B.B.s.

They also want 'scientific agreement' to determine what can be stated on your vitamin bottle. My answer would be: *"Just how would one go about agreeing scientifically?"* I presume it means having the agreement of scientists whom cooperate with them. In any event, it most certainly does not mean 'scientifically performed research' because that is what they seem to be fighting against.

Dr. Robert C. Atkins M.D, was the controversial founder and medical director of The Atkins Center, a world renowned integrative medicine practice located in Manhattan and author of *New Diet Revolution,* and *Vita-Nutrient Solution.*

The following is an excerpt from Dr. Newbold's book, Mega-Nutrients for your nerves: *"Too many of us in the medical profession feel too insecure to accept information tendered by our patients, fearing that our prestige might suffer if we do not appear omniscient. This is a great mistake. An intelligent and observant patient can often be of tremendous help to the doctor, sometimes even when it comes to making a relatively simple diagnosis."*

Closed mind? Unable to learn new information? Have to be the expert exclusive of personal limitations?

I've met and worked with a lot of medical professionals, both as clients and in consulting with them, about their own health and fitness concerns, including health providers whom, seemingly out of insecurity in the own personality, come across like they have to be the expert in everything...they simply can't take in critical information that supplements what they learned or read in their initial training and education. They'll insist they want my help and expertise, then go out of their way to alter, dismiss, change, substitute or ignore what is suggested.

Especially in the medical-sciences, new information is emerging every day. But, people whom have to think of themselves as 'the' expert can't seem to take in the very information their body needs to maintain itself, not even considering how much the information would help their own patients. Did you get that gem there?

People whom are compelled to present themselves, as the expert, will argue indefinitely about every minutia of detail (to boost their ego) while their body continues to deteriorate from lack of the B.N.B.B.s. I refer to this as mental masturbation; *lots of talk and nothing produced.* Ironically, the more and longer the person has gone without adequate nutrition-density the less their pre-frontal cortex seems to function and the less able they are to monitor their own thoughts and behaviors and the less likely they are to recognize true, helpful, relevant information...in other words, they argue against the very information their body and brain requires, but their ego prevents the information from getting in and being recognized (emotionally-based reactions), rooted in nutritional inadequacy.

I have met medical professionals that have an underlying belief that no matter what someone says, they believe it's their *duty* to argue and debate. With all the new information and developments, it's nearly impossible for a full-time medical professional to keep up with all the latest research-developments.

In these cases, I simply bless them, say a silent prayer for them and send them on their way. I see my 'job' as to provide the most accurate and up to date information, which I actually apply myself. When I run into people (even if they are medical professionals) whom don't have a way to know real information from misleading hype and advertising there's really nothing else I can do for them. They have to put the information to work for themselves (put the B.N.B.B.s in their body and *let nature do the rest)*. I've worked with medical professionals whom are not getting the results they want using products they market themselves, yet they continue to use because they are effectively buying them from themselves.

There are so many people whom have been waiting, searching and praying for these solutions. I simply don't have the time to waste with contrary, polarizing-personalities and neither do they. If medical professionals have a patient whom shows up to simply talk about what they insist they 'know', aren't there to learn, are not responsive to professional-suggestions and/or are non-compliant, more often than not they are referred on...there simply isn't enough hours in the day to see everyone and that's part of why it can take months to get an appointment with any specialist...screening out the people whom are not ready to accept help or change as a person in order to heal. Think of it this way....*stop doing what hurts the health and do more of what builds health!*

One of my specialties is designing dietary-supplement programs for individuals, couples and families. I work with people whom have decided they want the benefits I talk about in here and are ready to be shown exactly what to do. If someone just wants to debate and argue I simply don't have time for them...until they are ready to take suggestions and act on them (follow through/do their part). With every client interaction, there's the part I do and the part the client has to do. Talking about nutrition is not going to help anyone...*it's in the doing (put the B.N.B.B.s in and let nature do the rest)*. The people whom thrive on knowing every single detail before they will be convinced are missing the point; you get remarkable results by putting nutrition in your body...*not from a feeling of knowing everything.*

There are those people whom seem to be addicted to information (ask question after question to delay/procrastinate action and personal responsibility), and after decades of this work my radar spots these personalities a-mile-away...and that's how far I stay away from them, too. The person whom is an information addict mistakes 'knowing more and more' for 'doing correct action'...information is power only when it's applied! I help people whom are ready to go and just want to be shown how to get results.

Supplements may improve teenage behavior in school:

Oxford researchers found that giving nutrition-supplements to teenagers may improve behavior in schools, writes Annie-Rose Harrison-Dunn, 23-Nov-2015.

Published in 2003, a study about teens' use of dietary-supplements they were asked the reasons why they take dietary-supplements. *Consumption of nutritional-supplements among adolescents: usage and perceived benefits by* Jennifer A. O'Dea.

Below are the responses teens gave, for why they supplement their daily, intake of Whole-foods with supplements.

- *"Keeps me healthy."*

- *"Iron, because I'm vegetarian."*

- *"Keeps me fit for sports."*

- *"Vitamin C to prevent colds."*

- *"Keeps your sugar levels up."*

- *"They taste yummy."*

- *"Mom gives them to me."*

- *"They are good for you."*

- *"Feel like you are doing something good for yourself."*

- *"I don't get enough fresh foods."*

- *"Vitamin C for the immune system."*

- *"Helps me to grow."*

- *"Quench thirst."*

- *"Give me more energy for sports."*

- *"Mom gives it to me."*

- *"Stops my cold sores."*

- *"To not get sick."*

- *"Helps me do better at sports."*

- *"For colds."*

- *"To stop me from getting sick."*

- *To help with my obesity—Mum gives it to me."*

- *"Don't know – Mum gives it to me."*

- *"Gives me energy."*

- *"Mum takes it for energy–she gives me one sometimes."*

- *"To build muscle tissue when working with weights."*

- *"Helps with weight training."*

- *"My brother gives it to me in a milkshake to build my muscles."*

- *"Had it because I was thirsty."*

- *"Tastes nice."*

- *"The energy gives you a lift."*

- *"There are lots of vitamins in it."*

- *"It was the only drink available."*

- *"Stops me getting cramps at sport."*

- *"It's just like a soft drink"*

- *"Cools you down."*

- *"Coach makes us drink it."*

- *"Gives you energy."*

- *"Makes your muscles relax."*

- *"Makes me feel more energetic."*

- *"Other guys in the team take it."*

- *"I don't think it does anything for me."*

- *"I had it because I was thirsty."*

- *"Wakes you up, makes you feel alert and it tastes nice."*

- *"I only bought it because there was no water."*

- *"It makes me go hyper."*

- *"I drink it before soccer, and I don't lose energy as fast."*

- *"I like the can—it looked cool, so I bought it."*

- *"They're like a soft drink."*

Some vitamins aren't good for you!

GreenMed Info posted an article in, May 2013, regarding toxins in children's vitamins: *Top Pharma-Brand of Children's Vitamins Contains Aspartame, GMOs, & Other Hazardous Chemicals.*

The #1 Children's Vitamin Brand, in the U.S., contains ingredients that most parents would never intentionally expose their children to, so why aren't more opting for healthier alternatives?

Kids vitamins are supposed to be healthy, right? Well then, what's going on with Flintstones™ Vitamins, which proudly claims to be, *"Pediatricians' #1 Choice."* Produced by the global pharmaceutical corporation Bayer, this wildly successful brand features a shocking list of unhealthy ingredients, including:

- Sorbitol

- Aspartame

- Zinc Oxide

- Cupric Oxide

- Ferrous Fumarate

- Sodium-Benzoate

- GMO Corn starch

- Hydrogenated Oil (Soybean)

- Coal tar artificial coloring agents (FD&C Blue #2, Red #40, Yellow #6) [made from the sludge left over after the production of gasoline].

On Bayer Health Science's Flintstones product page designed for healthcare professionals they lead into the product description with the following tidbit of information:

82% of kids aren't eating all of their veggies. Without enough vegetables, kids may not be getting all of the nutrients they need.

References: 1. Lorson BA, Melgar-Quinonez HR, Taylor CA. *Correlates of fruit and vegetable intakes in US children.* J Am Diet Assoc. 2009;109(3):474-478.

The implication? That Flintstones™ Vitamins somehow fill this nutritional void. But let's look a little closer at some of these presumably healthy ingredients....

Aspartame:

Aspartame is a synthetic combination of the amino acids aspartic acid and l-phenylalanine, and is known to convert into highly toxic methanol and formaldehyde in the body. Aspartame

198

has been linked to over 40-adverse health effects in the biomedical literature, and has been shown to exhibit both neurotoxicity and carcinogenicity. What business does a chemical like this have doing in a children's vitamin, especially when non-toxic, non-synthetic non-nutritive sweeteners like stevia already exist?

Cupric oxide:

Next, let's look closer at Cupric Oxide, 2 mg of which is included in each serving of Flinstone's Complete™ Chewable Vitamins as a presumably 'nutritional' source of 'copper,' supplying *"100% of the Daily Value"* (Ages 4+), according to Flintstones™ Vitamins Web site's Nutritional Info.

But what is Cupric Oxide? A nutrient or a chemical?

According to the European Union's Dangerous Substance Directive, one of the main EU laws concerning chemical safety, Cupric Oxide is listed as a hazardous substance, classified as both *"Harmful"* (XN) and *"Dangerous for the environment"* (N). Consider that it has industrial applications as a pigment in ceramics, and as a chemical in the production of rayon fabric and dry cell batteries. In may be technically correct to call it a mineral, but should it be listed as a nutrient in a children's vitamin? I think not.

Coal-tar based, artificial coloring agents:

A well-known side effect of using synthetic dyes is attention-deficit, hyperactivity disorder. There is also indication that the neurotoxicity of artificial food coloring agents increases when combined with aspartame, making the combination of ingredients in Flintstones™ even more concerning.

Zinc oxide:

Each serving of Flintstone's Complete™ Chewable vitamins contain 12 mg of Zinc oxide, which the manufacturer claims they deliver 75% of the Daily Value to children 2-to-3 years of age. Widely used as a sun protection factor (SPF) in sunscreens,

The EU's Dangerous Substance Directive classifies it as an environmental Hazard, *"Dangerous for the environment (N)."* How it can be dangerous to the environment, but not for humans ingesting it, escapes me. One thing is for sure, if one is to ingest supplemental Zinc, or market it for use by children, it makes much more sense using a form that is organically bound (i.e. 'chelated') to an amino acid like glycine, as it will be more bioavailable and less toxic.

Sorbitol:

Sorbitol is a synthetic sugar substitute which is classified as a sugar alcohol. It can be argued that it has no place in the human diet, much less in a children. The ingestion of higher amounts, have been linked to gastrointestinal disturbances from abdominal pain to more serious conditions such as irritable bowel syndrome.

Ferrous Fumarate:

The one clear warning on the Flinstone's™ Web site concerns this chemical. While it is near impossible to die from consuming Iron from food, e.g. spinach, Ferrous Fumarate is an industrial mineral and not found in nature as food. In fact, Ferrous Fumarate is so toxic that accidental overdose of products containing this form is, *"...a leading cause of fatal poisoning, in children under 6 years of age."*

The manufacturer further warns:

Keep this product out of reach of children. In case of accidental overdose, call a doctor or poison control center immediately.

Sodium-Benzoate

Why is sodium benzoate bad for you?

When sodium benzoate combines with Ascorbic Acid (Vitamin C), benzene can form, which is a known carcinogen.

Hydrogenated Soy Bean Oil:

Finding hydrogenated oil in anything marketed to children is absolutely unacceptable. These semi-synthetic fatty-acids incorporate into our tissues and have been linked to over a dozen adverse health effects, from coronary artery *dis*-ease to cancer, violent behavior to fatty-liver *dis*-ease.

GMO Corn Starch:

While it can be argued that the amount of GMO corn starch in this product is negligible, even irrelevant, we disagree. It is important to hold accountable brands that refuse to label their products honestly, especially when they contain ingredients that have been produced through genetic-modification. The 'Vitamin C' listed as Ascorbic Acid in Flintstones™ is likely also produced from GMO corn. Let's remember that Bayer's Ag-biotech division, Bayer CropScience, poured $381,600 of cash into defeating the Proposition-37 GMO-labeling Bill, in California. Parents have a right to protect their children against the well-known dangers of genetically-modified-foods and the agrichemicals that contaminate them, don't they? GMO corn starch is GMO, plain and simple. We'd appreciate it if Bayer would label their "vitamins" accordingly.

In summary, Bayer's Flintstone's™ vitamin brand is far from a natural product, and the consumer should be aware of the unintended, adverse health effects that may occur as a result of using it.

None of the B.N.B.B.s I recommend or personally use contain any of the above ingredients, either in children's or adult formulas. B.N.B.B.s refers exclusively to whole-food concentrates.

Feedamerica.org published the following statistics related to malnourished children:

Good nutrition, particularly in the first three-years of life, is important for establishing a good foundation that has implications for a child's future physical and mental health, academic-achievement, and economic productivity. Unfortunately, food-insecurity is an obstacle that threatens that critical foundation. According to the United States Department of Agriculture (USDA), 13.1-million children, under 18, in the United States live in households where they are unable to consistently access enough nutritious food necessary for a healthy life. Although food-insecurity is harmful to any individual, it can be particularly devastating among children due to their increased vulnerability and the potential for long-term consequences.

Food-insecurity:

• 13.1-million children lived in food-insecure households in 2015.

• 20% or more of the child population in 30-states and D.C. lived in food-insecure households in 2014, according to the most recent data available. Mississippi (27%) and New Mexico (27%) had the highest rates of children in households, without consistent access to food.

• In 2014, the top-five states, with the highest rate of food-insecure children, under 18, were Mississippi, New Mexico, Arizona, Alabama, and Arkansas.

• In 2014, the top-five states with the lowest rate of food-insecure children, under 18, were North Dakota, Massachusetts, Minnesota, New Hampshire, and Virginia.

Mariana Cares Mobile Unified School District Mobile Food Bus, for all school breaks, said Crystal Kalahar

• Proper nutrition is vital to the growth and development of children. While almost all (94%) of client households with school-aged children (ages 5-18) report participating in the National School Lunch Program, only 46% report participating in the School Breakfast Program.

• Nearly 1-in-4 (24%) client households, with children report participation in the Special Supplemental Nutrition Program for Women, Infants, and Children (WIC).

• ½ of client households that reported doubling-up (housing more than one family in the same living space) in the past 12-months have one-or-more children that are five-years old or younger.

• The majority (53%) of client households that are unstably housed (such as a shelter) have one-or-more children that are five-years old or younger.

Poverty Statistics:

• In 2015, 14.5 million or approximately 20% of children in the U.S. lived in poverty.

Participation in Federal Nutrition Programs:

• In fiscal year 2014, more than 20-million or 44% of all SNAP participants, were children under age 18.

• During the 2014 federal fiscal year, 21.7-million low-income children received free or reduced-price meals daily through the National School Lunch Program. Unfortunately, in 2014 fewer than 4-million children participated daily in the Summer Food Service Program and the Seamless Summer Option.

Infancy & Development:

Children growing up in food-insecure families are vulnerable to poor health and stunted development, from the earliest stages of life.

• Pregnant women whom experience food insecurity are more likely to experience birth complications, than women whom are food secure.

• Inadequate access to food during pregnancy has been shown to increase the risk for low birth weight, in babies.

• Food insecurity has also been linked with delayed development, poorer attachment, and learning difficulties in the first two-years of life.

Health Concerns:

Studies have found that food-insecurity has been associated with health problems for children that may hinder their ability to function normally and participate fully in school and other activities.

● Children whom are food-insecure are more likely to require hospitalization.

● Children whom are food-insecure may be at higher risk for chronic health conditions, such as anemia and asthma.

● Children whom are food-insecure may have more frequent instances of oral health problems.

● Food-insecurity among young children is associated with poorer physical quality of life, which may prevent them from fully engaging in daily activities such as school and social interaction with peers.

Behavioral Challenges:

Children whom experience food-insecurity may be at higher risk for behavioral issues and social difficulties.

● Food-insecure children may be at greater risk of truancy and school-tardiness.

● When they are in school, children whom are food-insecure may experiences increases in an array of behavior problems including: fighting, hyperactivity, aggression, anxiety, mood swings, and bullying.

● 1-in-5 US children do not have enough to eat.

The Guardian reported in their article entitled, *Hidden hunger: America's growing malnutrition epidemic,* **"...that even people in the wealthiest countries aren't getting enough nutrients,"** writes Barbara Bush, daughter of former U.S. President George W. Bush, and Hugh Welsh, President of DSM North

America. Some 85% of Americans lack essential vitamins. The word "hunger" calls to mind thin, starving children in developing countries, but in the U.S. today, the real picture of under-nutrition is different **(fat, but under-nourished)**. In some cases, children whom are obese whom are malnourished because they are consuming the wrong types of foods – *foods that are calorie dense, but nutritionally poor*. It is called "hidden-hunger" and it robs billions-of-people the opportunity to reach their full potential.

(I've read other studies that showed that even as income levels increase people end up consuming greater quantities of meats and calorie-rich foods, but still don't get enough B.N.B.B.s (nutrition-density)). Calories vs nutrients.

With hidden-hunger, officially known as micronutrient-deficiency, **(people eat enough calories, but fail to get essential-nutrients, such as vitamins and minerals)**. It's a well-recognized issue in developing countries, where organizations like the World Food Programme and many others work tirelessly to ensure that people – particularly young children – get the essential nutrition they need to reach their full physical and cognitive potential.

Babies are highly vulnerable to micronutrient-deficiency, up-to-age-two, (window of nutritional opportunity and requirements), when they are in a period of intense physical, motor and cognitive growth. *There is no way to catch up later.* Without that initial nutrition, children often deal with physical and mental deficits for the rest of their lives. Under-nourished-children are also more likely to suffer from illnesses, and as a result, less likely to perform well in school.

While awareness of malnutrition in the developing world is high, micronutrient-deficiency is rarely discussed in the US. However, it is a serious and growing challenge in all segments of our population, particularly among those with low and middle incomes, whom have limited access to – or simply can't afford – the perceived extra cost of essential-nutrition.

About 85% of Americans do not consume the US Food and Drug Administration's recommended daily intakes of the most important vitamins and minerals necessary for proper physical and mental development.

More than 1/2 of American children do not get enough of Vitamins D and E, while more than 1/4 do not get enough Calcium, Magnesium or Vitamin A, according to a recent *Journal of Nutrition* study. This can result in a compromised immune system, stunted physical growth, reduced mental ability, chronic *dis*-ease and even death. Magnesium alone is responsible for more than 300 different required actions in the body to maintain health.

The Centers for Disease and Control and Prevention reported August 5, 2014 in their article entitled, *Children eating more fruit, but fruit and vegetable intake still too low* that U.S. children aged 2-to-18 years are eating more Whole-fruit, according to the latest Vital Signs report by the Centers for Disease Control and Prevention. The amount of Whole-fruit consumed each day increased by 67%, from 2003 to 2010, but is still low. Vegetable intake was also low and remained unchanged, during the same time period.

From 2003-2010, the amount of fruit-juice children drank decreased by about 30%, and Whole-fruit replaced fruit juice, as the main contributor of fruit to children's diets. Experts recommend that the majority of fruit come from Whole-fruit, rather than juice.

Despite this progress in fruit intake, children still fail to meet recommendations for the amount of both fruit and vegetables they should eat daily. 60% of children did not eat enough fruit to meet daily recommendations in 2007-2010, and 93% of children didn't eat enough vegetables. Recommendations for the amount of fruit and vegetables children should eat are based on a child's age, gender and level of physical activity. Recommendations range from 1-to-2 cups for fruit and 1-to-3 cups for vegetables.

CNN reported in their article dated November 23, 2011, *1-in-5 U.S. children at risk of hunger*. The number of families that struggle to get enough food has increased in recent years. The U.S.

Department of Agriculture reported that in 2010, 14.5% of households in the United States -- about 17.2-million -- lacked the resources to provide enough food for everybody. Among those, about 6.4-million households saw normal eating patterns disrupted or reduced because there wasn't enough food. They're likely to have trouble focusing in school. They might experience illness or poor health as a result. They're also likely to struggle with stress at home or in class. While many are eligible for free or reduced-price food at school, those programs don't provide food at night, on weekends or during breaks from school. Hunger is still a more frequent problem for homes headed by single parents and for homes below the federal poverty line, the USDA reports, but it has also crept into homes that have never experienced it before.

Bill Moyers reported on April 5, 2013 in an article entitled *Going to Bed Hungry,* that poorly-nourished children have lower school test scores and require far more long-term health care spending. Hunger also reduces the productivity of workers, which reduces their earnings, which, in turn, reduces their ability to purchase nutritious-food for their children. In this vicious cycle, malnourished-children do not do as well in school, are more likely to drop out, and are less likely to go to college than children whom are properly nourished. **Consequently, malnourished-children earn less as adults and are less able to help America build a 21st-century high-skills economy.** In order for the nation to build the best public education system in the world, bring down health care costs, and rebuild our economy, we simply must reduce lack of nutrition-density in the diets. Hunger in the world's wealthiest nation is not only morally-unacceptable, it also costs the U.S. economy at least $167.5-billion per year, in large part because of its negative impact on children, according to the Center for American Progress.

PRI.org reported on January 28, 2016 in their article *Why Are Kids Going Hungry in One of California's Most Productive Farming Regions?* That makes the next statistic even more startling: the percentage of children going hungry in Imperial Valley ranks among the worst 10% of all US counties.

Imperial County has the highest rate of child hunger in the entire state of California, with close to 40% of kids not getting enough food. The majority of the county — more than 80% — is Hispanic.

Persistently low wages, unstable employment and severe drought conditions have taken a major toll on local agricultural workers and their families. And, that's hitting young people the hardest.

The Washington Post reported on March 9, 2017 in their article *Reading, writing and hunger: "More than 13-million kids in this country go to school hungry."*

DoSomething.org, a global movement of 5.5-million young people reported that in their research, they found that:

● 1-in-6 people in America face hunger: The USDA defines "food-insecurity" as the lack of access, at times, to enough food for all household members. In 2011, households with children reported a significantly higher food-insecurity rate, than households without children: 20.6% vs. 12.2%.

● Food insecurity exists in every county in America. In 2013, 17.5-million households were food-insecure. More and more people are relying on food banks and pantries. Collect food outside your local supermarket for a local food bank. Sign up for Supermarket Stakeout GL.

● 49-million Americans struggle to put food on the table. In the US, hunger isn't caused by a lack of food, but rather the continued prevalence of poverty.

● More than 1-in-5 children is at risk of hunger. Among African-Americans and Latinos, it's 1-in-3.

● Over 20-million children receive free or reduced-price lunch each school day. Less than 1/2 of them get breakfast, and only 10% have access to summer meal sites.

● For every 100 school lunch programs, there are only 87 breakfast sites and just 36 summer food programs.

● 1-in-7 people are enrolled in Supplemental Nutrition Assistance Program (SNAP). Nearly 1/2 of them are children.

● 40% of food is thrown out in the US every year, or about $165-billion-worth. All of this uneaten food could feed 25-million Americans.

Sooooo, where are all the people whom are getting enough nutrition whom are 'healthy' and eating a 'balanced' diet?

Chapter Twelve

Choosing Good B.N.B.B.s

There are basically three-types of nutritional supplements on the market. Two of them will leave you wondering *"What happened?"* or *"Why aren't I getting the kind of results Sov said I would?"*

The 3rd and worst/unhealthiest kind of dietary-supplement will likely get you *more* than you bargained for:

● Synthetic or test tube vitamins:

● Based on the philosophy, 'more is better'/quantity versus quality.

● Known as *pharmacy*, pharmaceutical, physician's, medical or prescription-grade.

● Ingredients are man-made in a laboratory.

● Derived from petroleum and coal tar *(the sludgy stuff left over after the production of gasoline...literally!)*.

● Can be irritating to the tissues, causing sores and cracks in the mouth, gastrointestinal upset, nausea and headaches to name a few reactions and side-effects and they do not feed the cells.

● Stimulate the cells without feeding them.

(That would be like if you visited my office because you wanted more energy and before you sat down, I had wired the chair to shock you and make you jump up! When you sit down on it, you suddenly jump up, without even thinking about it. That is what stimulants do to the body. They force the cells to work even though the energy/nutrition supply may be exhausted).

• Under a microscope, the shape or structure "resembles" vitamins, but they are biologically-<u>in</u>active, especially so compared to the B.N.B.B.s.

• I have never heard of anyone experiencing any benefits from these, although they are the most readily available prescribed at the doctor's office, grocery store, big box stores, pharmacy, nutrition stores and discount suppliers.

Trying to identify vitamins as single chemical structures is short-sighted because you have to have the entire complex to get the benefits nature intends. Since the prescription drugs merely cover up problems while they continue to gain momentum inside the body, it's no wonder the same chemists try to 'take-nature-out-of-nature' and market/advertise fake/synthetic vitamins as the real deal.

Note: On my blog, I have several articles that go into greater detail including pictures and examples of where chemicals that are considered toxic, national, manmade-disasters, as well as toxic-contamination to spawning salmon are being used to manufacture synthetic vitamins, also known as prescription grade, naturopathic grade, pharmaceutical grade, vegetarian, vegan, GMO free, drug store variety, big-box store variety, discount vitamins and food-based dietary-supplements...*it's ridiculous*. These 'vitamins' are 'irritating' to the cells of the body to say the least. You can access my blog here:

https://sovereign-valentine.mykajabi.com/

Dr. Theron G. Randolph, MD, wrote in his book, *Human Ecology and Susceptibility to the Chemical Environment*, *"A synthetically-derived substance may cause a reaction in a chemically susceptible person when the same material of origin is tolerated, despite the two substances having identical chemical structures. This point is illustrated by the frequency of clinical reactions to synthetic vitamins – when these naturally occurring vitamins are tolerated. There is also other evidence indicating that the biological activity of synthetic and natural vitamins is not identical."*

I am afraid the effect this has on everyone's state of health and wellness is massive. The S.A.D.C.R.A.P. has relied upon the processing of food and then enriching and fortifying it, after the fact adding only a fraction of the original vitamin content and to top it off, the food companies replace the lost nutrients with synthetic ones. Flour for instance has more than thirty-nutrients removed, then four-or-five are replaced with synthetic ones, while the stuff that is removed is fed to livestock to increase profit.

The first commercially processed flour showed up in 1905. That is when the good stuff began being removed. By 1912, the term 'heart-failure' showed up in the medical literature. Until then, there was not even a term for 'sudden-death'. In 1939 federal law required food processors to add back [four of the 25-to-30 removed B.N.B.B.s].

People along the way throughout history whom tried to stop this process, even top government officials were undermined and ran over by profit hungry business people whom influenced government with their money...*in other words, there is a lot of money at stake that influences public health policy.*

By 1920, the epidemic of heart *dis*-ease was gaining momentum. Today, heart *dis*-ease is the number-one killer competing with obesity...both results of lack of the B.N.B.B.s.

Get it? The B.N.B.B.s are removed to prevent spoilage and extend shelf life of S.A.D.C.R.A.P. so food companies can control profit better for stock shareholders. Nutrition is removed from food the same way precious metals are removed from the soil. Then the nutrition is sold to feed animals. Then the nutritionally-void food is marketed and sold as nutritionally-rich. In essence, so they can predict profitability of their companies. The removed B.N.B.B.s are called 'mill-feed' and they are marketed and fed to livestock which are raised for profit. The animals get fed what people are supposed to, so they can have optimal muscle (meat) before being slaughtered.

Removal of the B.N.B.B.s deludes the ability of the body, [every system and capability], to consistently maintain, repair, rebuild, recover and perform at peak-levels. The stuff added back into the food is synthetic, made from petroleum (coal tar). When the body shows signs of wear and deterioration, the doctors may prescribe drugs made of other toxic chemicals to cover up the symptoms, so we really do not know what's happening to the body...the underlying lack of nutrition-density goes on...that's your responsibility to put the B.N.B.B.s back into your body.

Even though this has been going on for nearly a hundred-years, it's a 'medical mystery' because in some cases the so-called medical experts are funded by the people whom control the food, the drugs **and** the information about how toxic their food and drugs are and how much nutrition is missing from the food supply.

Each new child that is born, can expect to have a level of health determined by the number of generations born to their family whom have eaten S.A.D.C.R.A.P. as a result of some health providers saying, *"Nutrition does not have anything to do with your health."*

Profit? The Center for Science in the Public Interest, *Nutrition Action*, (Vol 16, No 1) reported that, *"...the only difference between General Mills' Wheaties and Total cereals is that 1.5 cents worth of vitamins are sprayed back onto Total cereal." Total* is then sold for 65 cents more than *Wheaties and the nutrition removed is sold to livestock producers, to keep those animals healthy!*. This practice alone generated $425,000,000.00 in additional profits for General Mills...**in 1972!!**

The Surgeon General's Report on Nutrition and Health 1988 said, "All pharmacological therapies induce side-effects [pharmacology has been described by part of the scientific community as "applied toxicology" because even the desirable effects of drugs are obtained by altering-poisoning normal metabolic function], and high-dose nutritional-therapies are no exception." All drugs by definition are poison and abnormally high potency vitamin supplements are drugs. (Only the synthetic vitamins achieve this drug status).

J.I. Rodale, The American Naturalist, wrote in his book, *The Complete Book of Food and Nutrition*: *"We must take vitamins if we wish to be healthy and the nation as a whole must do it, or God alone knows what will happen to the second-or-third generation coming up-generations inheriting weaknesses passed on to them by us, generations which few of us will live to see unless we augment our diet with vitamins and minerals. And as parting advice, do not take coal tar [synthetic] vitamins. Be sure the vitamins you take are from food. Scientific research proves that this is best."*

The 2nd-type of dietary-supplements are called:

- Extracted or crystalline vitamins:

- Based on the philosophy, *"People won't know the difference."*

- Typical health food and grocery store variety.

- Often referred to as 'food-based' or 'vegetarian-formula' because the synthetic vitamins are combined with some food like rice bran or alfalfa.

- Incomplete...may be from food but missing many important keys to health like the enzymes, bioflavenoids, life-force, phytochemicals.

- Unknown/un-named components are left out or destroyed in the packaging process.

- Contain binders, fillers, artificial coloring and other unnecessary chemicals.

- Heat and or chemical like solvents (hexane for example, which is basically gasoline) to strip the vitamins out of the food. Many important factors are destroyed in the process. Then the hexane is burned off, leaving only the "skeleton" of the original nutrients.

- Can cause side-effects like indigestion, headaches, nausea and whom knows what else.

• The cells of the body use up energy trying to break these two-types of vitamins down in the body and get little, if anything in return. You take vitamins to get energy and the body wastes energy trying to make energy? Makes sense, right? Maybe not cents, but dollars, *for the companies*. These extracted vitamins are marketed/advertised as natural and health-building, but they aren't capable of producing the results they imply.

Poopy?

I have met a few people whom work in the municipal water treatment plants and they tell me they see hundreds of vitamins floating in the untreated sewer water every day. Synthetic and extracted supplements simply don't even breakdown in the body. I have seen X-rays of people's large intestines, with synthetic or extracted vitamin-supplements that are getting ready to pass out of the body un-dissolved.

The producers of these types of vitamin-supplements arrogantly behave as if they know all the functions and intentions of nature.

The 1st kind of dietary-supplement and where you want your attention to be and where you actually get more value than you pay for:

B.N.B.B.s:

Based on the philosophy of *"Building health by feeding the cells what they need."*

• They are as close to nature as possible.

• Contain the known and unknown factors.

• Contain the fractions that have not even been named yet (because they aren't destroyed).

• They have strong enzyme action, thereby enhancing the body's inherent health-building actions (that is like a fresh set of spark plugs or a freshly charged battery!).

• Processed in low heat, low pressure with no chemical solvents.... to preserve the life-force of the food.

• Highest quality raw food materials.

• Based on nature's standards...not man's standards.

• Feeds the cells... rather than poking fun at them.

• Dissolve within 15-minutes, after entering the body.

• Startling results. This is why people call me and say, *"Sov, you won't believe what happened...thank you so much!"*

• Nature can't be built in after the fact...quality comes from not destroying what nature created.

• Some people whom ego consider themselves experts will still say, *"There's no difference."*

Compare apples and oranges to petroleum. Which would you rather eat?

It is unnecessary to sacrifice safety and effectiveness, but many manufactures still do it.

The best of science and the best of nature.

Next are some excerpts from an article which ran on April 17, 2000 by The PR Newswire and *a Seattle newspaper:*

The National Academy of Sciences says, *"The various forms of Vitamin E need to be reevaluated to determine their relative strength and make labels more understandable."*

"Vitamin E in capsule form, from soybeans (concentrated food), has been found to be twice-as-effective, as synthetic versions from petroleum-products."

"Vitamin E from soybeans is called <u>d</u>-alpha. The synthetic version is called <u>dl</u>-alpha. Additionally, Vitamin E from food can fall into any of eight different categories." (Can be called eight different names and contain eight different beneficial-types of Vitamin E).

"Nutritionists said, "...estimates of Vitamin E are difficult to make and there are insufficient distinctions (among supplement companies), among types of E."

"Most nutrition data bases, as well as nutrition labels do not distinguish among different types. Data is often measured in the form of alpha-tocopherol equivalents." (The real food form, yet the marketing and distribution of synthetic versions refer to the standards of food-concentrate level/quality Vitamin E to support the use of synthetic Vitamin E).

"Because the various forms of Vitamin E are not inter-convertible, it is recommended that relative biological potencies of the various forms of E be reevaluated and researchers should report separately on actual concentrations of each of the various Vitamin E forms."

In other words, Vitamin E in food concentrate form (B.N.B.B.s), is twice as effective as synthetic Vitamin E. Vitamin E from food is what the people and books in the nutrition-industry are referring to when they say how much to consume, but synthetic supplement manufacturers make cheaper, less potent and less effective forms out of waste petroleum-products and measure and label it as if it were from food...they are not making distinctions between synthetic and food concentrates and they do not convert the same in the body. Then, consumers wanting the most for their money are mis-lead, when comparing prices of synthetics and extracted to food concentrates (bait-and-switch).

That is one of the **Reasons** you may have n*ot r*eceived **Results** before.

How about you?

Would you say there is a difference?

If you have supplemented your diet with dietary-supplements of any kind in the past and got minimal or no results, or even negative side-effects, here are just a few potential reasons why...

• *The Los Angeles Times* ran a story about having 10 brands of St John's Wort, a popular herb used for depression, tested. 7-out-of-10 had less key ingredients than promised on the label. 3 had less than 50% of what was promised on the label.

• A study mentioned in *The New York Times* revealed that 60% of certain pure herbal supplements were so watered down that they were worthless.

• Consumer Labs, tested 30-brands of Ginko Biloba, a popular herb for memory and concentration, in August 1999. 25% had less key ingredients than promised on the label.

• Consumer Labs, tested 27-brands of Saw Palmetto, a popular herb for the prostate gland in men, in December 1999. Ten had less than the required beneficial ingredients. One had zero beneficial ingredients.

• Consumer Labs, tested 13-brands of SAM-E (S-adenosyl-methionene) in March 2000. Six had as much as 50% less than the label promised.

• Consumer Labs, tested 35-brands of calcium, in August 2000. 4 contained less than the label. One had 53%, one had 61%, one had 82% and one had 91% of what the label promised.

• Consumer Labs, tested 22-brands of Ginseng, one of the most widely used herbal supplements in the world. 2, had 20-times the allowable amount of quintozene and or hexachlorobenzene (known poisons). Two had high lead content and 7 had less than the required concentration, of the active part of the plant.

• Dr. Bob Doster, whom has worked in the food industry for years, tested 14-brands of B-Complex supplements right off the store shelves. 11 of them did not contain what the label stated and or failed to be absorbable by the body.

• He also tested 63-different acidophilus (*Pro*-biotics/the good bacteria found in our intestines) supplements. Only 5% contained the amount of good bacteria the label claimed.

• *Dallas Magazine* had 40-products from 5 different stores independently tested. 50% did not meet label claims. 5 had no active ingredients at all. Whole-foods™ Store brand had streptococcus bacteria in the pills.

Store Manager, Casey Rose, of Fresh Market™ at Oak Lawn in Dallas said, *"I have a lot of confidence in Solgar™ (brand) since they have been in business since 1947... there are a whole lot of reasons why I like them... they do not take short cuts in the manufacturing... they're the Cadillac of the vitamin industry".* ...In the testing, Solgar™ performed the worst of all.

The following is an excerpt from an article in *a* Seattle newspaper, Sunday March 19, 2000: *"In 1998, California investigators found that nearly 1/3 of 260 herbal products contained lead, mercury and or diabetes drugs that were not listed on the label."*

• Pediatrician Hillary Perr reported on children from wealthy California families whom became mal-nourished from eating snack foods that contained herbs. (The herbs, acting as stimulants to the body caused the bodies of the children to use up nutrients, leaving them mal-nourished after eating the "healthy snacks").

• In 1999, GHB, (gamma-hydroxybutyrate) a body building supplement was responsible for 3 Florida Poison Control Centers logging 549 negative incidences and 2 deaths. The same year the

FDA threatened lawsuits and search and seizure. One year later, with reports even higher, Congress outlawed GHB. There have been 60 deaths reported from GHB so far.

- Rexall Sundown's St. John's Wort herbal formula had only 20% of the labeled potency. In addition, Rexall used a legitimate company's peer-reviewed research work to support the claims for their product, which didn't come close to the quality of the research they were promoting.

- AP Newswire, October 26, 1999. Olathe, Kansas. A high school football player collapsed on the field after consuming 'Ripped Fuel' a dietary herbal supplement containing Ma Huang.

- A vitamin-supplement was recalled that contained Folic Acid, which women take to reduce the chances of having a baby with birth defects, because it contained only 35% of the amount claimed on the label, leaving the unborn child susceptible to spinal cord defects from Folic Acid deficiency

- The April 2000 issue of *Emergency Medicine* reported about a 30-year old athlete whom took androstenedione, a testosterone precursor. Touted as an "enhancer of athletic performance", his friend told him, *"Those pills will help build muscle size."* He took it for 7-days and by the time he was admitted to the emergency room he had been suffering for more than 30-hours with a painful, persistent erection. If untreated, tissue damage could have resulted. This condition is known as priapism.

- *Women's Sport and Fitness Magazine* ran an article entitled, *Brave New Foods*. Jed Fahey, research associate at John Hopkins University School of Medicine tested 20-brands of SGS (sulforphane glucosinolate) a known anti-tumor agent found in broccoli. 15-of-the-20 contained either no SGS or far less than the label claimed.

You see, there is very little regulation of the dietary-supplement market.

John C. Reed, an Arlington, Virginia physician and Vice President of Media Affairs for American Wholehealth says, *"...even if they correctly label it, it doesn't mean healthy bacteria actually end up living in your gut."*

Drugs, chemicals and contaminated products can be on the market for years, even when they are causing deaths before the companies or those responsible are shut down or products are pulled from the shelves.

Basically, anything can be labeled as a dietary-supplement and until there is proof that the product has been dangerous to many, many people, *business continues*.

Labeling of dietary-supplements often indicates, incorrectly, that they meet standards set by the United States Pharmacopoeia. **However, the United States Pharmacopoeia does not verify that products bearing the USP designation meet their standards of quality, and that includes promises made about ingredients listed on the label.** Most of the dietary-supplement companies in existence today are nothing more than marketing and advertising companies. They have nothing to do with building health.

This is how they work: They figure out their target market, say... 'weight-loss' or 'body building' then they hire a dietary-supplement bottling company to put their label with *implied* benefits on the bottle. And then they start selling them. They are not necessarily effective or safe, there is very little regulation and too few people to enforce the laws that are in existence.

You see, The Dietary-Supplement Act allows legitimate companies to share the facts about their products, but it also allows the dishonest people time to make a ton of money until they are shut down. It is a buyer-beware market. I have literally heard of companies that first figure out how high their risk of losing a liability lawsuit is.

Then they figure out how much profit is at stake. Last on their priority list is public safety. The way they look at is the very worst that can happen is that they will be forced to close their business, then they just open up under a different name.

By using certain supplements, you can have more energy and at the same time be doing damage to your body. Nervous system stimulant herbal formulas are in this category.

Although it took me about 10-years of experimenting on myself and thousands-of-dollars invested in some mediocre and some horrible supplements, the list below is what I have identified as criteria for quality food-supplements. B.N.B.B.s should [not], but more often than not have:

- Bacteria,

- Fertilizer,

- Pesticides,

- Hormones,

- Fungicides,

- False claims,

- Bactericides,

- Heavy metals,

- Misleading labels,

- Artificial coloring,

- Excessive potency,

- Artificial flavoring,

- Growth regulators,

- Unnecessary fillers,

- Artificial sweeteners,

• Unnecessary binders,

• Prescription and recreational drugs and/or

• Solvent extraction processing (using gasoline-like substances to pull the vitamins out of the Whole-food).

Unfortunately for us consumers, I have found in the 30-or-so-years I've been doing this stuff, that most of the supplements available have at least 2-or-3 of each of these no-no's. Its near impossible for the average consumer to know a good supplement from a poor-quality supplement and often even the sales person doesn't know the difference regardless what they say. It took me 12-years of constant research to find the truth about supplement quality and research has to go all the way to the corporate level to find the truth about supplements, even when they are marketed as healthy, natural, vegetarian, vegan, gluten free, GMO-free, organic and so on.

Although some of these sound a little ridiculous, you can find these things in any of the doctor's office vitamins, grocery store, health food store, drug store and pharmaceutical grade supplements, as well as some of the door to door varieties.

Special Note:

For those of you whom have purchased a copy of this book, and you want my help getting your program dialed-in you can contact me directly by my email which I've provided in the appendix of this book and I'll be happy to provide you a complimentary hour consultation by phone. I have very high standards for the B.N.B.B.s I use and am happy to share my favorites with my clients. After 30-years, I have enough confidence in my skills and experience that I can guarantee results and satisfaction. If you want to be shown exactly what to do, email me. I look for people whom are willing to give my suggestions a one-year commitment. It takes about a year to rebuild the entire body from-the-inside-out and I don't want you to miss out on any benefits. *If this describes you, I can't wait to talk with you.*

Here are a couple of preliminary tests you can do at home:

Reason 64. Pre-heat your oven to 350 degrees.

Place your Multi-vitamin tablet on a piece of aluminum foil and cook it for 10-to-15 minutes. Then remove it from the oven, do not touch it yet, and let it cool down. The stuff you see exuding from the vitamin is usually the binders, fillers, sugars, colorings and petroleum products. Not very scientific, but it lets you know what your body has to process.

Reason 65. Place your Multi-vitamin in a glass of water.

Then just let it sit. The USP standard is that a Multi-vitamin must dissolve in 30-minutes or less, in order for your body to have any chance of utilizing the nutrients. And remember, just because it dissolves does not mean it contains the basic nutritional building blocks in concentrated-food form.

This one is not scientific, either. The stomach should be more acidic which would make it dissolve even faster. People whom are healthy have enough live enzymes and acid to dissolve a supplement. People whom have not been following these guidelines often have a sluggish digestive system.

I would love to hear what experiences you have with these tests. Drop me a note in the mail of the products you test. I'll look forward to hearing from you! Please include the type (e.g., Multi-vitamin tablet, brand name and how much the supplement cost you).

One of the most popular vitamins available at most grocery stores didn't dissolve at all. When the manufacturers found out people were doing this test, they formulated their vitamin to dissolve, even though it is a synthetic vitamin made out of petroleum by-products.

Many times, the outside coloring or shell will fall off and the inside never dissolves.

When I say, *"It doesn't dissolve,"* I mean it goes right through your body without breaking down. As I said earlier, I have spoken with people whom work at city water treatment plants. They can see the vitamin tablets floating through the sewers with the actual name of the supplement still imprinted on it. Many of them!

When I was managing the GNC store, I tested every supplement that was returned. Some were still un-dissolved days later. These were some of the most expensive and most advertised products that are still on the market today.

Often manufacturers will put their stuff in gel-caps, so they dissolve very fast. That is very common with products marketed as vegetarian or food-based. That simply means the filler material is alfalfa or rice. They still fill them up with synthetic materials.

According to government standards, supplements labeled as 'natural' have to have only 10% of their ingredients as natural.

Reason 66. Travel?

If you've spent any time traveling you know that eating nutritiously is difficult enough when you're at home, have your resources available and are in your routine where you have access to your favorite foods. Traveling increases the need to supplement because quality of food is questionable and it's hit-and-miss. When you're traveling, sensible-supplementation is a convenient and cost effective way to fill in the gaps, cover your bases and help prevent illness while on the road.

Reason 67. Food Desert?

A food desert, as defined in *Webster's Dictionary* is an urban area where it is difficult to buy affordable, quality, fresh food. In other words, all around the country there are neighborhoods where the local convenience stores stock the affordable and convenient S.A.D.C.R.A.P, but fresh, nutrient-dense foods simply aren't available. In many such neighborhoods, residents don't have cars that they could use to go pick up groceries so their reliance on low nutrient-dense foods and beverages is high and residents end up malnourished, behavioral problems are high, relationship difficulties are higher, violence and crime is high...poverty reigns. Research has shown that behavior, ability to think and reason and ability to focus and stay out of trouble and simply get alone with others is more difficult the higher the rate of under-nourishment.

Michelle Miller on Los Angeles, CBS news reported on March 5, 2017 that *Food Desert Residents:*

- Weigh more,

- Suffer from higher rates of *dis*-ease like diabetes and

- Have a shorter life expectancy.

Chapter Thirteen

ENOUGH!!!? huH? "dOn'T i GEt eNOUgh frOM fOod?"

A lot of people (including myself) whom have practical-experience with nutrition think that the government nutrition standards are too low, for many outcomes.

In my experience (being considered generally healthy, having multiple chronic symptoms and even when I was sick and didn't feel good at all), I needed higher levels of Vitamin-C Complex, to stop the bruising and nosebleeds. I needed higher levels of Beta Carotene to make the insane dry-eye itching associated as hay fever to subside. I needed supplemental *Pro*-biotics to get my digestive system to calm down. I seemed to need higher levels of the Vitamin B-Complex to not feel fatigued all the time. Upon entering kindergarten, I needed extra Iron since my diet was so limited and the digestive problems, from consuming such high amounts of high fructose corn syrup interrupted my digestion, so much that I can only speculate this compounded the disruption in vitamin absorption and exacerbated too few natural enzymes from excessive processed foods. I seemed to be lacking some enzymes that assist with digestion and absorption, as when I began supplementing, I began gaining lean mass at an astonishing rate compared to a high calorie routine (6,000 calories/day).

Even during all these health problems the registered dieticians I sought help from insisted that since I was "fairly healthy" and I generally eat a balanced diet, I probably got enough nutrition from the food I was eating and shouldn't need supplements. Thank-goodness I trusted my gut, went and got the information I needed and ultimately got more relief than I needed.

Have you heard a dietician say, *"As long as we are "fairly" healthy and generally eat a balanced diet, we shouldn't need to take supplements?"* Another peculiar thing is that many of these dieticians take supplements *themselves*...so, knowing how to eat isn't the answer even for dieticians.

One study, https://nutritionj.biomedcentral.com, reported 74% of 300 dietitians surveyed said they were regular users of dietary-supplements. The primary reasons for using dietary-supplements were:

● For bone health (58%),

● Overall health and wellness (53%) and

● To fill nutrient gaps (42%).

Of the ones whom personally use supplements and subsequently recommend patients take supplements said the reason for recommending them are, *"...there are gaps in clients' diets that could effectively be addressed with dietary-supplements."* Of the 300 dietitians surveyed 96% said they also followed healthy habits, including eating a 'balanced diet'.

Nearly all respondents (95%) expressed an interest in continuing education about dietary-supplements, on a variety of topics.

In my research over the last 30+ years, **I have found that not one single group of people gets even the minimum amount of nutrition every day, neither children, adolescents, adults nor seniors are getting the minimum amount of nutrition to even prevent the outward signs of malnutrition.**

Generally, impoverished people tend to lack quantity of nourishing food, yet people for whom socio-economic status is improved, tend to eat foods rich in meat and fat, but still lack nutrition-density (quantity does not equate to quality of nutrition-density). In June 2014, one study showed only 20% of school age children get their minimum amounts of nutrition on a daily basis.

To compound the issue, many things either increase the need of nutrient-density of the body and/or decrease the absorption of nutrients...*IF the nutrients are even there to begin with!!!!*

Personally, I don't know anyone whom eats perfectly all the time, so to me, supplementing makes good sense and assures you'll at least get the minimums met.

An article is posted on:

http://www.eatright.org/resource/food/vitamins-and-supplements/dietary-supplements/vitamins-minerals-and-supplementsv, reviewed by Sharon Denny, MS, RDN, Published January 07, 2016, entitled *Vitamins, Minerals and Supplements: Do You Need to Take Them?*

In addition, if you are eating less than 1,600 calories each day because you are trying to lose weight, you have a poor appetite or you have trouble eating because you have been using alcohol or drugs, discuss the need for supplements

Some individuals are limited in their food choices due to allergies, a medical condition or because they are following a vegetarian or vegan diet. For example, animal-based foods are the main source of Vitamin B12, so people whom follow a vegan diet need to eat fortified foods and/or take a supplement.

So, these organizations tend to say only these special groups of people need to supplement as if they don't know how many people are in those groups whom they themselves recommends they supplement.

Whom eats right all the time?

Whom eats all their meals every day?

Whom doesn't have special requirements...the question really is, *"Whom doesn't need supplemental B.N.B.B.s?!!"*

Eatright.org goes onto to say, *"Women whom are at an age where they could become pregnant need to obtain adequate Folic Acid, from fortified foods (cereals and other grains), supplements or both, in addition to consuming Folate from foods in a varied diet. Because it helps reduce the risk of some birth defects, Folic Acid is very important during childbearing years."*

Vitamin D might be a concern among infants, children and young adults. Infants whom are breast-fed and children whom consume less than the recommended amount of Vitamin D fortified milk or formula and those with increased risk of deficiency will likely need supplemental Vitamin D. Adolescent girls, often, might need additional Iron.

On the other side of the spectrum, as people age it can be difficult to get enough Vitamins B12 and D. Luckily, this is one of the cases where supplements can make a difference. Getting B12 from fortified-foods or taking it alone or as part of a Multi-vitamin/mineral can help raise B12 in your blood. If you're taking calcium or a Multi-vitamin, try to pick one up that also has Vitamin D.

Other groups whom may require additional supplementation include people whom are taking certain medications or have a health condition that changes how their body uses nutrients, and individuals whom have been told by their doctor they have a specific nutrient-deficiency.

The National Institute of Health says:

"Women need Iron during pregnancy, and breastfed infants need Vitamin D. Folic Acid, whether from supplements or fortified food is important for all women of childbearing age."

Research suggests that fish oil can promote heart health. Of the supplements not derived from vitamins and minerals, Hopp says, *"Fish oil probably has the most scientific evidence to support its use."*

National Institute of Health says:

"Just because a supplement is promoted as 'natural' doesn't necessarily mean it's safe. *The herbs Comfrey and Kava, for example, can seriously damage the liver."*

Personally, I focus on eating 1) Whole-foods 2) Functional-foods and 3) some B.N.B.B.s, to make up for nutritional-gaps.

Part of what took me more than a decade to learn was how to define standards for high quality B.N.B.B.s that the *good* manufactures use and the ones most neglected by marketing companies masquerading as "health" companies. As you read through these you are likely to understand why the average consumer or sales-person isn't going to go to the trouble to find all this stuff out. In a lot of cases, supplement companies that don't have high standards simply don't respond to inquires, from consumers...*why might that be?*

The National Institute of Health says, *"It's important to know the chemical makeup, how it's prepared, and how it works in the body—especially for herbs, but also for nutrients,"* says Carol Haggans, MS, RD.

Manufacturers are also responsible for the product's purity, and they must accurately list ingredients and their amounts. **But there's no regulatory agency that makes sure that labels match what's in the bottles.** You risk getting less, or sometimes more, of the listed ingredients. All of the ingredients may not even be listed.

A few independent organizations conduct quality tests of supplements and offer seals of approval. This doesn't guarantee the product works or is safe; it just assures the product was properly made and contains the listed ingredients.

The National Institute of Health says, *"More than 1/2 of all Americans take one or more dietary-supplements daily or on occasion. People take these supplements to make sure they get enough essential nutrients and to maintain or improve their health."*

Haggans, a registered dietitian and consultant to The National Institute of Health said, *"But supplements can be useful for filling in gaps in your diet."* ***Evidence does suggest that some supplements can enhance health in different ways.*** The most popular nutrient supplements are Multi-vitamins, Calcium and Vitamins B, C and D. Calcium supports bone health, and Vitamin D helps the body absorb Calcium. Vitamins C and E are antioxidants; molecules that prevent cell damage and help to maintain health.

On the FDA website:

https://www.fda.gov/Food/ResourcesForYou/Consumers/ucm1097 60.htm an article is posted, *"Whom is responsible for the safety of dietary-supplements"*

FDA is *not* authorized to review dietary-supplement products for safety and effectiveness, before they are marketed.

The manufacturers and distributors of dietary-supplements are responsible for making sure their products are safe, BEFORE they go to market.

If the dietary-supplement contains a NEW ingredient, manufacturers are *supposed* to notify FDA about that ingredient prior to marketing. However, the notification will only be reviewed by FDA (not approved) and only for safety, not effectiveness.

Manufacturers are required to produce dietary-supplements in a quality manner and ensure that they do not contain contaminants or impurities, and are accurately labeled according to current Good Manufacturing Practice (CGMP) and labeling regulations.

If a serious problem associated with a dietary-supplement occurs, manufacturers are supposed to voluntarily report it to FDA as an adverse event. FDA can take dietary-supplements off the market if they are found to be unsafe or if the claims on the products are false and misleading.

Part of what I have done for the last decades, is help people make good decisions about getting their B.N.B.B.s program started and dialing-in their current nutrition program. Once you've read this book, you can contact me at the email shown in the appendix and for your complimentary, one-hour consultation.

Below is a partial list of some of the things that tend to increase the need for nutrition of the body, above the minimum government standards. ***When you have two-or-more of them combined, there's not likely a chance you're even coming close to getting what you need nutritionally, without some supplementation.***

Testing by the manufacturer of dietary-supplements to assure safety and effectiveness should include:

1) ***A genuine need by the body for the product.***

One of my favorite pet-peeves is when the molecular biology of some part of the body is studied at a microscopic level. The people doing the study find some enzyme, chemical or whatever that exists at some point in the process of living. Often the particular chemical is a product of several physiological steps of metabolism. Then they learn to make the chemical synthetically, in the lab, and market it as the newest weight-loss or muscle-building formula. People rush out to get it, by the time the truth is found out the company has made ten-million-dollars and has gone out of business.

2) ***Clinical proof via independent, double-blind, placebo controlled and randomized studies on human volunteers, with the final results published in peer-reviewed major medical journals...*not pseudo-science information or advertisement magazines.**

Companies often claim to have done studies on their products. It means nothing. The kind of studies I describe above are done in such a way that nobody involved in the study, neither the participants nor the organizers of the study can control or manipulate the outcome of the study.

Sometimes, like Rexall™ did, that I mentioned earlier, use results of good studies done by other companies as the basis for their product. And they'll even go so far as to say, *"See, it is proven to work."* Only problem is Rexall's product was almost empty of the ingredients needed to get the benefits that the study referred to. This practice is so common I cannot even believe it.

3) A report from the supplier.

Of the raw materials, to the supplement producer regarding the cleanliness of the raw materials and the contaminants that were tested for by the supplier.

4) The producer of the supplement should *retest the raw materials:*

To confirm or disclose discrepancies in the raw material supplier's report. Certified-Organic Food simply refers to food up until the time it is harvested. **Often the raw materials that are Certified-Organic get exposed to toxins *after* being harvested, packaged and shipped to distributors or consumers.** So conscientious B.N.B.B. producers test the raw materials to find out if they have been exposed to toxins following harvest or during transport.

5) Finished products should be *tested rigorously for contaminants, potency and bioavailability*.

In other words, the product needs to be checked to see if anything got mixed in that was not supposed to. Then checked to see if the amounts in the product match what the label claims. Then the product needs to be tested to find out if the product makes its way into the bloodstream, where it can do its job.

6) Herbal raw materials and final products need to be *tested via high performance liquid chromatography* to determine the identity of the herb and the concentration of the important ingredients.

7) Herbal raw materials also need to be tested via thin- layer- chromatography to detect *substitutions or changes made, by the supplier of the raw materials*.

If the raw materials of the product are grown using pesticides, herbicides, fungicides and things like that the body sees the product as a toxin and gets rid of it instead of really making use of the nutrients in hopes of detoxifying the body…*the cells miss out and recovery is hampered.*

And more importantly, the producer/seller of the products should *guarantee the potency and bioavailability* of the product (*at the time*) you consume it. Bioavailability refers to whether or not the nutritional ingredients actually make it into the bloodstream. Often companies guarantee the potency only at the time the product was manufactured which basically eliminates any responsibility on their part and do not even take bioavailability into account

The products should have a *100% money back guarantee.* In other words, you buy the products, use them all up and if you are not satisfied you get all your money back. That's it. Anything less is questionable to say the least.

To give you some idea of how many supplement companies have the philosophical integrity to police themselves and build a product based on a genuine desire to help people build their health I offer you this example.

Dr. Bruce Miller, speaker and author of *Nutrition Guarantee* and numerous other nutrition related books, videos and audios contacted over 220 different dietary-supplement companies, by registered mail over a 17-year period, inquiring about peer-reviewed studies done on their products. Only one did any real scientific research themselves.

In October 2001 Consumer Labs did an independent test on 30-different, sports-type nutrition bars. 18 did not meet the claims on the labels and half of the bars contained more carbohydrates than the labels stated. One label stated it contained two grams of carbohydrates when it actually contained 22-grams, so it is important to purchase products you know you can trust.

Dietary-supplements, which are not concentrated food-supplements (B.N.B.B.s), tend to work against each other, creating side-effects like nausea, headaches and other weird symptoms whereas the concentrated food-supplements work synergistically, enhancing each-others' properties.

Some scientists and politicians will say, *"...there is no benefit or difference in the types of dietary-supplements,"* but my experiences have demonstrated there are significant differences.

● **Nature can't be built in after the fact.** There is no tricking the body. Once the raw materials are damaged or contaminated during farming, harvesting, transporting, manufacturing and/or distribution, no company can make up for it with false labeling claims.

● Apples or petroleum...*which do you want to buy and eat?*

● The cells of the body need to be fed food for their loyal service...your health and performance is dependent on real nutrition-density getting into the cells of your body.

● Dietary-supplement companies should answer all your questions. Complete disclosure and show proof of their claims.

● **There are three-types of dietary-supplements. Some stimulate and exhaust the cells. Some nourish and feed the cells the basics so they can build optimal health and performance.**

● In other words, some supplements look 'ok' under the microscope, but the cells can tell the truth and it is reflected in the condition of the body's health and performance. Not by how people interpret what nature intended.

● There are thousands of dietary-supplements on the market. Some are safe, some are not. A thousand companies come and go every year. Often, consumer mistake "new" for better, but that's rarely the case.

● Focus on putting the B.N.B.B.s in your body and *let nature do the rest.*

• Athletes on a good nutrition program experience many unexpected side benefits.

• Our nutritional needs are as individual as our fingerprints.

• When we see or hear claims made by dietary-supplement representatives, ask for their double-blind, randomized, placebo controlled, clinical study results that were performed on human volunteers and published in peer-reviewed major medical journals, with their own products -*not a research referenced from a different company's products*. Also, ask if the company making the supplements will guarantee in writing to be free of:

• Pesticides

• Herbicides,

• Hormones,

• Fungicides,

• Artificial fats,

• Heavy metals,

• Heat processing,

• Mold and mildew,

• Artificial coloring,

• Solvent extraction,

• Growth regulators,

• Artificial flavoring,

• Synthetic fertilizers,

• Drugs and medications,

- Bactericides & bacteria,

- Misleading, hyped up labels and/or

- Unnecessary fillers and binders.

*Properly produced B.N.B.B.s are more clean, pure and more efficiently absorbed than Certified-Organically Grown food...*because the manufacturer tests the raw food materials before using them to produce the B.N.B.B.s.

Remember: USP certification is *not* a guarantee of quality, but a claim by the company.

To make it easy to find reliable information, NIH has fact sheets on dietary-supplements at: http://ods.od.nih.gov/factsheets/list-all/. NIH also recently launched an online Dietary-supplement Label Database at www.dsld.nlm.nih.gov. This free database lets you look up the ingredients of thousands of dietary-supplements. It includes information from the label on dosage, health claims and cautions.

The Federal Trade Commission posted an article entitled, *Tainted Products:*

In the last few years, FDA has discovered hundreds of 'dietary-supplements' containing drugs or other chemicals, particularly in products for weight-loss, sexual enhancement, or bodybuilding.

The 'extra ingredients' generally aren't listed on the label, but could cause serious side-effects or interact in dangerous ways with medicines or other supplements you're taking. People have suffered strokes, acute liver injury, kidney failure, and pulmonary embolisms (artery blockage in the lung); some people have died.

Tainted supplements often are sold with false and misleading claims like *'100% natural'* and *'safe'*. **Some things that help but are not conclusive in their own right** and to recognize tainted products, look for:

• Promises of rapid effects or results,

• Marketing materials primarily in a foreign language,

• Products claiming to be legal alternatives to anabolic steroids and/or

• Products claiming to be alternatives to FDA-approved drugs or have effects similar to prescription drugs.

Find more on tainted products marketed as dietary-supplements at the FDA's website.

The Federal Trade Commission posted the following article about dangerous supplements at:

https://www.consumer.ftc.gov/articles/0261-dietary-supplements#taintedproducts, written by Anahad O'Connor on October 14, 2015, entitled *Dietary-supplements Lead to 20,000 E.R. Visits Yearly, Study Finds:*

A large new study by the federal government found that injuries caused by poor quality dietary-supplements lead to more than 20,000 emergency room visits per year, many involving young adults with cardiovascular problems, after taking supplements marketed for weight-loss and energy enhancement.

The study is the first to document the extent of severe injuries and hospitalizations tied to dietary-supplements, a rapidly growing $32-billion-a-year industry that has attracted increased scrutiny in the past year and prompted calls for tougher regulation of herbal products.

Critics of the industry said that the findings provided further evidence that the relatively low level of regulation in the United States put many consumers at risk. But industry representatives said that the products were used by roughly 1/2 of all Americans and that the data showed only a tiny fraction sustained major injuries.

The new study was published in *The New England Journal of Medicine* and led by health authorities at the Food and Drug Administration and the Centers for Disease Control and Prevention. The researchers tracked emergency room visits at a large network of hospitals around the country over a 10-year period and then analyzed those in which a dietary-supplement was implicated.

Among the injuries cited were severe allergic reactions, heart trouble, nausea and vomiting, which were tied to a broad variety of supplements including herbal pills, amino acids, vitamins and minerals. Roughly 10% were serious enough to require hospitalization, the researchers found.

In comparison, prescription drugs are responsible for 30-times as many trips to the emergency room each year.

One finding was that emergency room visits caused by supplements occurred predominantly among young people, whereas those for pharmaceutical products occurred in large part among older adults, said Dr. Andrew Geller, a medical officer at the division of health care quality promotion at the C.D.C. and the lead author of the study. *"The contrast is striking,"* he said.

More than 1/4 of the emergency room visits occurred among people ages 20-to-34, and 1/2 of these cases were caused by a supplement that was marketed for weight-loss or energy enhancement, commonly producing symptoms like chest pain, heart palpitations and irregular heart rhythms.

These products typically contain a variety of herbs and extracts and are widely advertised online, in magazines and on television with names like Hydroxycut™, Xenadrine™, Raspberry Ketones™ and Black Jack Energy™, the researchers said.

It was unclear how many, if any, of these cases are fatal because the study tracked hospital visits, not deaths. Weight-loss supplements and energy boosters have been implicated in serious problems, including one outbreak in 2013 that sickened 97 people and caused at least one death and three liver transplants.

Under a 1994 federal law that has been widely criticized by health authorities, supplements are considered safe until proved otherwise. Unlike prescription drugs, they do not have to be approved by the F.D.A. before they are sold to consumers, nor are they required to list major side-effects.

"This is very disheartening," said Dr. Pieter Cohen, an assistant professor at Harvard Medical School whom was not involved in the new research. *"What we're seeing from this study is that the system has failed. It's failing to protect consumers from very serious harms."*

The study also pointed to other flaws in the regulations. The F.D.A., for example, recommends limits on the physical size of prescription drugs, but no such regulations exist for supplements. The new study found that about 1/3 of supplement-related emergency room visits, for people 65-and-older, were caused by choking on pills like Calcium and other vitamins and minerals. A large proportion also had allergic reactions.

But Duffy Mackay, a spokesman for the Council for Responsible Nutrition, a supplement industry trade group, said that, *"...if anything, the new research highlighted how relatively safe supplements are, given how many people took them."*

"We have over 150-million Americans taking these products each year," he said. *"This suggests that far less than 1/10th of 1% of supplement users will visit the emergency room."*

Mr. Mackay said that choking and other hazards highlighted by the study could be addressed by the F.D.A. *"If they think that capsule sizes in the elderly are an issue, they could put out an advisory and the industry would respond,"* he said. *"The current law as it's written has everything in it to make this change."*

Peter Lattman and Anahad O'Connor authored an article entitled, *Makers of Nutritional Supplements Charged in Federal Sweep* in November 2015.

A year-long federal investigation into the dietary-supplement industry has resulted in a widespread crackdown on the sale of tainted or misleading products.

The Justice Department said on Tuesday that it filed criminal and civil enforcement actions against 117-companies and individuals.

At the center of the sweep is USP Labs™, a company based in Dallas that sold the best-selling workout supplements Jack3d™ and OxyElite Pro™, which contains the amphetamine-like stimulant dimethylamylamine, or DMAA. On Tuesday, federal prosecutors brought criminal charges against USP Labs™ and six of its executives related to the sale of those products.

News of the crackdown caused the shares of the country's leading nutritional supplement retailers, including GNC™ Holdings and the Vitamin Shoppe™, to decline.

The indictment against USP Labs™, filed in Federal District Court in Dallas, accused the supplement manufacturer of telling its retailers and wholesalers that it used natural plant extracts in its products, when in fact it was using a synthetic stimulant made in a Chinese chemical factory.

According to the indictment, the use of OxyElite Pro™ led to a number of liver injuries, including at least one death.

Marketers said the supplements increased strength, speed and endurance, and they became popular with workout enthusiasts.

In December 2011, after the deaths of 2 soldiers, whom had used Jack3d™, the Defense Department removed all products containing DMAA from stores on military bases, including more than 100 shops operated by GNC™ Holdings, the nation's largest retailer of nutritional supplements.

In 2013, under pressure from the Food and Drug Administration, USP Labs™ voluntarily destroyed its inventory of Jack3d™ and OxyElite Pro™.

Among those arrested was Jacob E. Geissler, 39, the chief executive of USP Labs™, whom according to the company's defunct website, studied nutrition at Texas A&M. Mr. Geissler and USP Labs™ could not be reached for comment on Tuesday.

Shares of GNC™ Holdings, Vitamin Shoppe™ and other retailers that sell nutritional supplements dropped after the Justice Department announced midday Tuesday that it was holding a news conference to present the charges. Shares of GNC™ declined as much as 27%, and Vitamin Shoppe™ shares fell as much as 10%.

But after it became clear that the retailers were not being named in any of the cases, shares recovered. Still, at the close of trading, GNC™ had dropped 6.4% and Vitamin Shoppe was down 4.9%.

GNC™ has come under increased scrutiny over the last year. Last month, the Oregon attorney general sued the company, accusing it of selling dietary-supplements with illegal and dangerous ingredients. At the time, GNC™ said the claim was meritless.

And in March, GNC™ struck an agreement with the New York State attorney general to begin using sweeping new testing procedures on its herbal products.

The attorney general had accused GNC™ and three other retailers of selling herbal supplements that were fraudulent or contaminated with potentially dangerous ingredients.

In a statement Tuesday night, GNC™ said, "...*it had provided its full cooperation,*" to the authorities. The company said it was, "...*committed to maintaining the trust and confidence of our customers.*"

The Justice Department, which worked alongside the F.D.A. and other federal agencies in its investigation, said on Tuesday, "...*it had also filed complaints against numerous companies that have sold supplements as cures for dis-eases or that were otherwise in violation of the law.*"

The case against USP Labs comes as part of a broader crackdown on the supplement industry, which faces calls for tougher regulation of its products after a number of deaths and illnesses linked to them.

"The Justice Department and its federal partners have joined forces to bringing to justice companies and individuals whom profit from products that threaten consumer health," said Benjamin C. Mizer, principal deputy assistant attorney general, in a statement.

"The USP Labs™ case and others brought as part of this sweep illustrate alarming practices the department found," he said, *"...practices that must be brought to the public's attention, so consumers know the serious health risks of untested products."*

Published in April 2015, an article talks about some of the dangers of improperly formulated supplements: *Study finds amphetamine-like substance in diet pills, supplements:*

An amphetamine-like compound that has never been tested in humans is in a range of popular diet pills and sports supplements, a study in a pharmacological journal has found.

The substance, known as BMPEA, is found in products advertised as containing Acacia Rigidula, a shrub native to Texas. In fact, the study said, the compound can only be produced synthetically, is not listed on labels, and its health risks are unknown.

The study, published Tuesday in the journal *Drug Testing and Analysis*, said the Food and Drug Administration discovered the presence of BMPEA in dietary-supplements in 2013, but failed to warn consumers or order its removal.

Spokeswoman Julie Putnam acknowledged the agency published research on BMPEA found in Acacia Rigidula supplements in 2013.

"While our review of the available information on products containing BMPEA does not identify a specific safety concern at this

time, the FDA will consider taking regulatory action, as appropriate, to protect consumers," she said.

The manufacturer of Arco Black Series Burn™ said Monday it was pulling all products containing BMPEA from its website.

"While the FDA has not declared the fat-burning ingredient BMPEA to be harmful," said Kathleen Reed, an executive with Vitacost™, a Boca Raton, Fla., unit of grocery giant Kroger™, *"...we take safety concerns very seriously for all of the 45,000-plus products sold on Vitacost.com."*

The study is another round in a long-running battle among supplement makers, regulators and researchers over the safety and efficacy of dietary-supplements, which, under the 1994 Dietary-supplement Health and Education Act of 1994, are not subject to FDA testing before being brought to market.

With the FDA empowered to act only after problems are discovered, the result has been a cat-and-mouse game, in which researchers discover problems, regulators act, and supplement makers adjust their products and practices, only to start the process all over again.

In 2018, nutritional-supplements retailing giant GNC™ Holdings signed a settlement with New York Attorney General Eric Schneiderman requiring it to begin using DNA-based testing to authenticate the ingredients, in a series of herbal supplements.

The latest study — by Cohen, his Harvard Medical School colleague Clayton Bloszies, Caleb Yee of Haverford College, and Roy Gerona of the University of California, San Francisco — stems from research the FDA itself began, in 2012, on supplements featuring the Acacia Rigidula plant.

In a 2013 paper, the agency revealed the presence of a *"non-natural"* amphetamine-like substance, in 9-of-21 supplements tested.

The recent study tested 21-brands of Acacia Rigidula supplements and found BMPEA, in more than half of them. Among them were Jet Fuel Superb™rnv, Jet Fuel T-300™, Fastin-XR™, and other supplements made by Hi-Tech Pharmaceuticalsv, based in Norcross, Ga. The company did not immediately comment.

The study said research on dogs and cats from the 1930s and 1940s showed it to be associated with increased blood pressure and heart rate and that it is among the compounds banned by the World Anti-Doping Association.

On the other hand, the B.N.B.B.s I refer to contain _none_ of these questionable or harmful ingredients and are safe to use even by Olympic Athletes, whom constantly get tested for banned and dangerous ingredients. The B.N.B.B.s have never caused illness, injury or side-effects.

So, you can see that you have to be very careful when choosing supplements. According to the law, ingredients in supplements have to be shared with the FDA, but they don't have to be tested prior to hitting store shelves. Until people get sick or die, there's nothing else the FDA can do to protect you.

The following is another example of a pretty well-known company went too far and got in trouble.

Herbalife $200 million for false claims: (July 2016)

The Federal Trade Commission announced today that the diet and nutrition company Herbalife will have to pay a $200 million fine and restructure its business in response to allegations of *"unfair and deceptive practices."* ...The FTC called the settlement a *"significant law enforcement action."*

Caught on Video: Can Herbalife Cure a Brain Tumor?

Herbalife was the focus of a year-long ABC News investigation in 2014, in which two reporters went undercover as Herbalife recruits and found a company that has struggled to prevent distributors from embellishing the financial prospects of a sales career there and hyping the health benefits of its products.

ABC News found that nearly 600 independent distributors of the diet and nutrition sales brand Herbalife had been disciplined by the company in 2013, for making medical claims when selling the company's weight-loss shakes and supplements, despite company policies aimed at preventing such tactics.

In one instance, a Staten Island, N.Y., Herbalife distributor even told a potential customer -- whom was actually an ABC News reporter wearing a hidden camera -- that a woman with a brain tumor became symptom free after starting on Herbalife products.

"She used to shake like this because she lost control of her motor skills to the tumor and she said part of her cerebellum was deteriorated," he said. *"If you see her now, she's like one of us here...whatever it is that the product did, it helped her a lot."*

Herbalife executives told ABC News at the time that they were *"appalled"* by the investigation's findings and would take pains to prohibit such tactics. The company announced a *"significant re-training initiative."*

"In direct response to the interview where Brian Ross brought to light instances of members making unauthorized product claims, the company began a significant re-training initiative," Herbalife spokeswoman Barb Henderson said in an email then.

Herbalife officials today counted the settlement with the FTC, as well as a $3-million settlement with the Illinois Attorney General, as victories and claimed the settlements were *"an acknowledgement that [Herbalife's] business model is sound,"* in the words of Herbalife CEO Michael Johnson.

Essentially, the FTC and FDA found that Herbalife's business model was fine, but the distributors were making claims that went beyond what the law allows.

After being in the nutrition industry for decades combined with my personal-experiences, I'm completely confident in my ability to help you choose a safe dietary-supplement program that is safe and effective.

Athletes can also contact me to make sure the athletic supplements meet the requirements of the national and international competitive athletic rules as well as prevent violation of any of their laws.

Chapter Fourteen

The 10 most common mistakes people make with B.N.B.B.s:

1) Taking this information and trying to apply it, without guidance:

I simply can't believe it when folks can relate to the disappointment of using poor-quality supplements, seem to see the sense of feeding the cells with real food and then intent on applying these practices go to the local grocery store or their physician and buy synthetic or extracted supplements, *expecting to get the same results!* Buying poor-quality supplements or supplements touted as complete, prescription-grade and patting themselves on the back, yet doing the same things that have never worked before. A lot of the agencies insist people talk to their doctor about how to get on a good supplement program, but doctors don't get but a couple-hours of training in nutrition, unless they seek out nutrition training on their own, outside medical school, residency, or fellowships. If a doctor has good personal-experiences with dietary-supplements then they might be able to make recommendations, but if they don't have personal-experience, how can they make recommendations? And whom would you want guidance from, someone with decades of successful personal-experience or none at all?

I do think dietary-supplements should be readily available without medical help, but people whom would use 'not knowing how to start' as an excuse for not starting is unacceptable or getting poor quality supplements, just to be able to say they 'tried' it is irrational.

Solution: My email is in the back of the book and I'm happy to offer you a complimentary consultation and help you get started safely and properly, in order to maximize your results!

2) Asking for help and then not acting on it:

One of the Catch-22's of poor-nutrition is that lack of follow-through, on a proven concept. People whom are undernourished will invest time in appointments, pay the big bucks for the information and guidance and then analyze the information to the point that they never follow through on it in timely enough manner, for it to really help them the way they want it to (analysis-paralysis). In other words, one of the markers for an under-functioning upper brain is intellectualizing the idea of getting healthy and then not following through...*thinking that thinking is enough!* Why I got such good results is because I simply did what I was shown to do!

Solution: Ask me for help and then act on the suggestions you get.

3) Herbs in nutritional supplements:

One of the main points here that sets this information apart from the other stuff out there is that in order to have optimal health and get the most from your supplements, you have to first, feed the cells the *nutrition* they need as the base of improvement. As the health of the cells improves there is less reason to attempt to 'treat' conditions which are often from too little nutrition. There's a lot of Multi-vitamins on the market which are either synthetic or extracted and have little nutrition content, but then have an herbal concoction added to seemingly add value (bait-and-switch). I personally do use *some* herbal supplements, *but not in place of the B.N.B.B.s.* Get your B.N.B.B. program put in place, *first,* and then add herbs if you still think you need them.

Often, whence getting the guidelines about how to choose good B.N.B.B.s, people go and try to find the most sophisticated supplements they can. In short, they end up with supplements that are short on real nutrition and heavy in extra herbs and filler-ingredients, which are little more than sales-hype to make the customer think they are getting a lot of value in their purchasing decision... a lot of ingredients for which there is no proven use by the cells of the body, as well as quality control issues/contamination with any herbs that are supposedly added…and unnecessary added costs.

Truth is, that most herbs should only be taken to treat symptoms and if the dietary-supplements contain any herbs they have too little to make any difference medicinally, anyway…so, the customer ends up with a supplement short on the nutritional-B.N.B.B.s and short on the real nutrition, as well…a mediocre supplement at any price marketed as a higher ingredient product.

Solution: Ask me for help, act on the advice you get and make no substitutions or you'll compromise the information and your likelihood of getting the benefits I teach. If you want really good results, make use of the information I provide…*put it to the test!*

Solution: Avoid Multi-vitamins/minerals that include herbs. If there are herbs mixed in, you got shorted on the nutrition-density, itself. If you need to use herbs, get them separately to make sure they are full-potency and not an afterthought or as an attempt to create the illusion of 'added value'. There's not enough room in a vitamin tablet to add in extra ingredients, if the manufacturer is actually putting adequate nutrition-density in the tabs to begin with.

4) Chasing symptoms with individual supplements:

Once the body has begun to break down, mal-function, *dys*-function and/or *de*-generate into *dis*-ease it's simply too late to be messing around with individual-nutrients. The time for prevention has passed. Take all the B.N.B.B.s every day or you are wasting your time, energy and money and potentially compromising your choices for health in the future. If your primary goal is fat-loss, I have a specific program for that which will assist you in doing a one-eighty and begin to tour your situation around the very week we talk.

Solution: Instead of attempting to practice medicine and chase symptoms down with individual and/or high dose supplements, give your body a full spectrum foundation/base of the nutrition it definitely uses to build healthy cells and let nature take over. I think you'll be happy with the results...*in fact, I guarantee it.*

5) Relying on what you think, believe or wish were true:

We all wish we could get what we need from good, healthy food. Previous examples show this to be rare and inconvenient. Even I don't eat perfectly all the time, no one does.

Solution: Check yourself. Set your ego aside, it won't help you. What you 'feel' may not be reality. Put in what nature designed your cells to use and let nature take over. It's not uncommon for the people whom have the least amount of nutrition in their body (highest need in the brain) to pay attention to the emotional 'feelings' which ends up being over-functioning emotional areas of the brain, due to lower functioning pre-frontal cortex (from lack of nutrition-density). When the pre-frontal cortex (cooperative, cognitive, rational, goal setting, long-term goal accomplishing, recognition of truth & compassion, self-care), doesn't have enough nutrition-density, the brain tends to default to the limbic (emotional aspect of the brain), resulting in (un-cooperative, emotional, irrational, want-it-now, short-term, immediate satisfaction, inability to recognize truth & compassion, impulsive, hurry-up-and-wait, attraction to sugar and S.A.D.C.R.A.P). The body requires the B.N.B.B.s and often people don't know how bad they felt until they have provided their body what it needs nutritionally, even when their ego thought it would have no result.

"Human beings have a great capacity for sticking to false beliefs with great passion and tenacity."

— Bruce H. Lipton, *The Biology of Belief: Unleashing the Power of Consciousness, Matter and Miracles.*

6) Behaving as if they want to change the laws of nature; wanting to be an exception to the rules:

"Oh yay, that's real nice information, but what does that have to do with me?" If you're alive reading this, you need the B.N.B.B.s. That's it. You aren't an exception to any of it.

Solution: Put the B.N.B.B.s in and let nature take over.

7) Mental-masturbation:

People whom think being able to conversationally intellectualize how they don't believe in supplements or how they are an exception to the nutritional-laws-of-nature will get them more than just putting the B.N.B.B.s in their body and let nature take over...*a lack of faith in nature combined with an over-inflated sense of self.* In these cases, I just have to sit back, rub my head and think, *"Oh, wow...well, I'm just the messenger...I can't help everyone and I certainly won't do it for them let alone try to convince them."*

Some people have a chip on their shoulder. Some people have a defensive attitude. Some people have more to gain from being sick than healthy. Some people think they are smarty-pants. Some people hold higher value coming across as a smarter debater more important than taking care of their health...hey, more power to 'em...heck, its America you can pretty much do what you want!...succeed or fail, it's up to you. You have just as much right to fail as succeed.

Solution: Having an intellectual outlet is a good thing. But, if you think over-intellectualizing basic nutrition concepts will help you, your body and brain will miss out on the benefits of your body's dependency on fundamental nutrition...yes, the ego can get in the way of self-care. It happens all the time. I won't be able to help you, nor spend any time with you, but if that's where your satisfaction lies, more power to you.

8) Inconsistent consumption:

If you really want the benefits I talk about here, you have to take your B.N.B.B.s every day. Some vitamins are water-soluble. That means the body doesn't store them and you have to put them in with your morning and evening meals.

Solution: Be consistent.

9) Making exercise more of a priority than supplementing:

Big mistake. If you don't get a complete nutritional program 1) Whole-foods 2) Functional-foods and 3) the B.N.B.B.s designed for you, you'll likely not reach even your short-term goals, let alone sustain/maintain your progress. If you do reach your goal, ultimately, you'll reach a plateau where the body quits getting stronger and any body fat that gets burned off will start coming back on (about three-months in). If you do reach your goals, you won't be able to maintain your goals. That's what 20+ years professional experience…and another 20+ years of personal-experience has shown me. Most everything I teach and do correctly today is rooted in doing it incorrectly for the first 24-years of my life.

Solution: Figure out your primary goals for exercising and get a nutritional program designed for you. Ask me for help. Then do it.

10) A dismissive attitude:

Asking for help from an expert in their field, then not following through on the information.

Having your own ideas is an important part of being an autonomous human, but make sure you have an accurate way to discern the difference between having your own ideas and rationalizing self-destructive behavior you label as rational thinking. Believe me, I've seen it all and I'm not fooled or mistaken anymore.

Nutrition is a 'doing thing'. You're either doing it or you're not. If not, too bad for you. You're missing out. Talking is not doing.

Solution: As Army drill sergeants are known to say, "Pull your head outcha' two points of contact, Private!"

Chapter Fifteen

For men only...

Reason 68. Problems raising the flag?

Men's Health magazine asks, *"Want to have sex into your 80s? Start following these tips today: how to keep your private parts healthy,"*...pop supplemental [nutritional] insurance:

"If you aren't eating 2-to-3 servings of fatty fish per week, take two Omega-3 Fatty-acid supplements daily, EPA/DHA... as a kind of insurance policy."

Your medicine cabinet might be hurting you:

Certain antidepressants, blood pressure medications, narcotic pain relievers, and antihistamines can cause problems with your erection. But even over the counter meds might be causing you to droop. One of the most surprising culprits? Your allergy or cold medicine: *"The mechanism behind an erection is the exact opposite of having an adrenaline rush, and Sudafed™ acts very similar to epinephrine—the adrenaline hormone—killing any ability to get aroused,"* says Harry Fisch, M.D., Clinical Professor of Urology and Reproductive Medicine at Weill Cornell Medical College/New York Presbyterian Hospital, and author of *Size Matters*.

Men's Health says, *"Keep your gut in check."*

Straining your belt could put your penis at risk, too. Men with a waist circumference of 39-inches or greater are more than twice-as-likely to have erectile dysfunction, as those with waists below 35-inches.

Meaning, getting rid of the fat may very well improve sexual performance. A healthy fat loss program will help you do a one-eighty and get your lean body back as well as performance 'downstairs'.

For sexual health, *Men's Fitness* recommends some:

Vitamin D:

Researchers at Johns Hopkins University, last year, looked at 3,400 healthy Americans and found that men whom were Vitamin D deficient were 32% more likely to have trouble getting it up than those with sufficient levels, even after adjusting for other ED risk factors. In fact, the connection is so common, Walker says D levels are something he always checks in ED patients. Why? The sunshine vitamin is crucial for keeping the endothelial cells that line blood vessels healthy. Without enough of the stuff, blood flow is inhibited, affecting everything from your heart to your hard-on.

Remember reason #45? Lack of sunlight is a reason to add the B.N.B.B.s to your Whole-foods regime.

Niacin/B-Complex:

A daily dose of Niacin (one of the eight B-Complex vitamins), improves erectile function, particularly in men with high cholesterol, according to a 2011 study in *The Journal of Sexual Medicine*. The vitamin helps increase blood flow and reduce inflammation—one of the underlying causes of both high cholesterol and erectile dysfunction. *"Vitamin B3 is also used to make sex hormones and other important chemical-signal molecules,"* says Fisch. Like many of the others on our list, this tablet is most powerful when taken in conjunction with others...and niacin taken for 3-months improved 40% of erections in a study from researchers at Sapienza University of Rome, Italy.

B-Complex is one of the 7 B.N.B.B.s that when taken in combination provides better results than taken individually. B-complex is made up of 8 different B-vitamins.

Folic Acid/B-Complex:

A Turkish study last year found that men with moderate to severe ED had significantly lower levels of Folic Acid, than guys without the problem. The B-vitamin has been shown to stimulate nitric oxide, Walker says, which would explain why an absence of it would lead to an absence of an erection.

B-Complex is 8 vitamins that make up one of the 7 B.N.B.B.s, that when taken in combination provides better results than taken individually.

On the website *Eat this not that*, clear recommendations for the best supplements for the penis are provided. The website asks, *"Have you fed your penis today?"*

That's no joke. Like every part of the body, the male reproductive system needs the right nutrients for optimal health, from function to fertility. Studies have isolated several nutrients that are particularly beneficial...we've broken them down here by nutrient in case you want to ensure you're getting enough.

Zinc:

In the modern era, people with higher levels of Zinc in their system have been shown to have a higher sex drive, than those with lower levels. That's because the mineral is essential for testosterone production. In one study, Zinc-deficient men whom supplemented with Zinc, for 6-months, doubled their testosterone levels. And another 8-week trial found that college football players whom took a nightly Zinc supplement showed increased testosterone levels as well.

Personally, I find Zinc that does not contain added sugar to make the biggest difference.

B12/B-Complex:

This is one B-Team you want to get on pronto: A recent report from Harvard University highlighted a study that has linked low levels of B12 to erectile dysfunction. A causal link hasn't been nailed down, but the B-vitamin is used by every system in the body, particularly in cell metabolism and the production of blood, two essential factors in getting and keeping a quality erection.

Vitamin D:

The sunshine vitamin will brighten things up in the bedroom. In a recent study published in *The Journal of Sexual Medicine*, Italian researchers found that of 143 men with erectile dysfunction, 80% had less-than-optimal levels of D, and the men with severe ED had, on average, a 24% lower level of D than with a milder condition. They theorize that low levels of D damage blood vessels and lead to a shortage of nitric oxide (while helps with dilation of blood vessels at appropriate times).

Vitamin C-Complex:

Vitamin C-Complex has been associated with higher sperm counts. You can get it naturally from strawberries, raspberries and blueberries, which are anthocyanins, colorful plant chemicals which help keep your arteries unclogged, boosting circulation and erection quality. In supplement stores, you'll find all manner of mega doses — steer clear of those; they might do more harm than good.

Personally, I recommend a three-part nutrition program: 1) Whole-foods, 2) Functional-foods and 3) B.N.B.B.s. Mega-dosing can be dangerous, but appropriate levels for your current fitness level and health goals is a safe approach.

Magnesium:

A mineral involved in muscle development, muscle is essential for reproductive function, in men of every age and activity level. One study that compared athletes to non-active individuals, found that supplementing with 22 mg Magnesium, per-pound-of-body weight over the course of 4-weeks, raised testosterone levels in both groups. And two separate studies, one on a group of men over the age of 65 and a second on a younger 18-to-30 year-old cohort, present the same conclusion: levels of testosterone (and muscle strength) are directly correlated to the levels of Magnesium in the body.

Folic Acid/B-Complex

Keep your 'swimmers' in fighting-shape, with Folic Acid (otherwise known as Folate). A deficiency can cause an increase in sperm with chromosomal abnormalities. And one study showed that sub-fertile men, whom supplemented with Folic Acid (B-Complex) and Zinc experienced a 74% increase in sperm count.

Selenium/best when combined with Vitamin E-Complex:

Selenium, found in Brazil nuts, liver and oysters, is a trace mineral that plays an important role in hormone health. You only need a tiny bit for healthy sperm, but a tiny deficiency can be catastrophic for reproductive health. In one study, men whom had lower testosterone and were infertile also had significantly lower Selenium levels than the fertile group. Supplementing with the mineral improved chances of successful conception by 56%. And a second-study, that included 69 infertile men with low levels of the mineral, found Selenium supplementation could significantly improve sub-par sperm motility associated with testosterone deficiency.

Vitamin A:

A study published in the journal *Fertility and Sterility* that analyzed the effect of various fruit and vegetables on sperm quality discovered carrots had the best all-round results on sperm count and motility, a term used to describe the ability of sperm to swim towards an egg. Men whom ate the most carrots saw improved sperm performance by 6.5%-to-8%.

Niacin/B-Complex

When it comes to maintaining your libido, the B-Vitamins are all your wingmen, but Niacin (a.k.a. Vitamin B3) is especially helpful. In a study published in *The Journal of Sexual Health*, men suffering from impotence whom took a Niacin supplement reported a significant improvement in their bedroom performance than men whom took a placebo.

Vitamin E-Complex:

Vitamin E-Complex helps improve circulation, boost testosterone and has been associated with increased libido.

LiveStrong,com suggestions:

Science has identified a number of nutrients that are vital to the penis and all it can do. Four of those seem to be more helpful than others:

• Zinc boosts testosterone levels and helps enable erections and healthy sperm.

• A deficiency of Vitamin B12 has been linked to erectile dysfunction, Harvard researchers found. The vitamin is crucial to cell metabolism and the production of blood.

• Magnesium decreases inflammation in blood vessels, increasing blood flow, which speeds blood to extremities, increasing arousal, and …well, you get it.

• Complete proteins relax blood vessels and enables blood to flow, helping you get and keep an erection. Of course, protein not only builds the lean muscle that helps you end up in bed with company in the first place, it's the most basic building block of tissue, dense in the amino acids that promote sexual health. Aim for GMO-free protein, which doesn't contain hormone altering substances.

My suggestion:

94% of protein supplements contain some GMO ingredients, which potentially interfere in healthy hormone production, while about 6% are GMO-free and that's some of what I personally use and specialize in suggesting my clients put in their body. If you're attempting to get better performance out of your body, start by eliminating ingredients which interfere...*you'll be happy you did and feel the difference.*

Chapter Sixteen

Reason 69. *Epigenetics*

"We are not victims of our genes, but masters of our fates, able to create lives overflowing with peace, happiness, and love."

Bruce H. Lipton, *The Biology of Belief: Unleashing the Power of Consciousness, Matter and Miracles.*

As described on nature.com: *"Epigenetics involves genetic control by factors other than an individual's DNA sequence. Epigenetic changes can switch genes on or off and determine which proteins are transcribed."*

Nutrition falls under this classification as something [on the outside of the body] that once put in the body can affect the genes, by introducing those factors that left without, manifest as signs, symptoms, *dis*-ease, health problems, etc. In other words, genetic-health problems can remain asymptomatic or 'latent' (asleep/inactive/repressed), when the body gets enough quantity, quality and consistency of proper nutrition-density.

When people purposely withhold the B.N.B.B.s (for whatever reason they insist) the genetic-potentials are more likely to manifest (awaken/active/expressed), with symptoms, whereas they may not when they purposely put the B.N.B.B.s in the body, with consistent intention. In simple terms, adequate-nutrition (what I coined as the B.N.B.B.s), can provide the factors which the DNA/RNA uses to prevent unhealthy expression of genes or indirectly cause potential health problems/hereditary/genetics to remain [latent] -*'unexpressed' throughout life.*

To further explain, in as simple as possible terms, people whom have what they have been told are hereditary or genetic-conditions, bad luck or otherwise unavoidable health problems often find that when they get enough B.N.B.B.s for their particular body, health things they previously believed they had to live with simply become less intense or go away completely, for no apparent reason thereby improving overall quality of life and performance, but return once inadequate-nutrition is inadvertently skipped or purposely discontinued.

There's a ton of ongoing controversy on these kinds of topics, partly because each school of thought or profession has their own standards (which not everyone agrees on), as well as informational biases that their profession adheres to. In other words, if you come from the world of treating *dis*-ease, there's the potential bias that information about preventing genetic *dis*-ease is invalid. Even in professional realms, people don't know what they don't know and would rather avoid giving any advice than advise they aren't sure of, which is responsible. For example, I read one study done at Children's Hospital, Seattle that showed that unless a doctor or nurse has had success with what is considered adjunctive-modalities they don't share the information with their patients.

Because nutrition in general is misunderstood, even by health professionals, I've found there's more *mis*-information than valid information available and being shared, within professional-realms and among consumers...*too much opinion and not enough correct application.* There's a lot of money made from fake, bogus, contaminated, hyped-up products that don't do anything good for the body.

One of my specialties is to train people to get on a sensible, dietary-supplement program to make up for inherent gaps in their daily nutrition-habits.

Even people whom know really well how to eat good don't get consistent nutrition day-in and day-out...*knowing how you should eat is not the same as getting enough nutrition in your body.* People whom know the most about nutrition take supplements even though they do eat really well, every day, leaving nothing to chance...*no stone unturned.* If you leave stones unturned, your priorities might be mixed up and I would refer you to my other book again. This is a doing program, not a saying or talking about program...*doing.*

People whom insist they want to achieve higher levels of health and performance, but withhold the B.N.B.B.s may need to consider their priorities...*the differences between what they say they want and what actions they do.*

A person who insists they want to lose weight, but also insist their reasons are more important than their results have just discovered the reason they haven't lost or kept weight off before!

When there is inner-conflict, a person may insist they want peak performance, to feel better, get leaner but spend money on coffee, ice cream, liquor and so forth, while purposely resisting the B.N.B.B.s...**it's very common for people to mistake 'talking' about nutrition as applying nutrition and then insist they don't know why they aren't feeling better or improving...(denial).**

Some professionals say you don't have to get enough nutrition daily (that the averages over a period of time are enough for everyone), but in my experience, rather than having an 'opinion' or an 'idea' (regardless of professional status) **body composition improvements and blood chemistry lab results are the two most accurate, science-based ways to know if you're consuming enough nutrition,** as well as whether or not what you're consuming is getting onto your blood stream and into the cells where nutrition actually does its job...**putting food or supplements in your mouth and swallowing them does not assure they're working** (a reason why there's so much misunderstanding and mixed results with dietary-supplements).

The point being that you can sidestep genetic, hereditary as well as health problems caused by medical treatment that could have been avoided. If you are bleeding or having any other type of emergency you should go to the emergency room immediately. But, a large portion of the reasons why people go to the emergency room (some doctors say about 90%) is from conditions caused by lifestyle-factors (lack of proper exercise and nutrition), which evolve into chronic health conditions and ultimately become acute, emergency health conditions.

Case in point: Alberto Salazar:

Coach of *Nike Oregon Project*, American Track Coach, world-class distance runner, author.

Alberto Salazar, author of *Alberto Salazar's Guide to Running* and *14-Minutes: A Running Legend's Life and Death and Life*, started out as a high school stand and was a state cross country champion, in 1975. From there, he went to the University of Oregon where he won numerous All American honors, was a member of the 1977 NCAA cross country championship team, won the individual NCAA cross country championship in 1978, finished third in the Olympic trial 10,000-meter race, to make the 1980 Olympic team. Alberto broke the 5,000-meter record in February 1981, at the Millrose Games in New York. His 13:22.6 beating the old record by nearly 20-seconds, as he finished second.

From 1980-1982 Salazar won three consecutive New York City Marathons. Alberto excelled at distances from two-miles, to the 54-mile length of Africa's Comrades Marathon, which he won in 1994 (the year the course went up hill)...*an amazing athlete to say the least.*

At age 48 (June 30, 2007) and 158 pounds (144 being his competition weight) and approximately 5% body fat/still lean and running 25-30 miles a week, running six-days-a-week, Alberto stopped breathing and dropped to the ground, at the Nike Training Center in Oregon. *"They had to shock my heart four-times, before they finally got my pulse back, which was 13-to-14 minutes after I first went down,"* said Salazar...*"Within an hour they placed a stent in a major artery."*

Prior, his doctor had noticed his blood pressure had been on the upswing for about a dozen-years, running about 140/97 and lowering to about 125/75 on medication (average normal would be about 120/80). Alberto was also taking cholesterol medication, which lowered his total cholesterol to about 175.

Alberto had a complete physical a couple-months prior to the event. He had seen his general practitioner, whom was a really fit runner herself and had kept his health in check. Alberto even had an EKG performed and everything checked out fine, but he did have some family-history of heart *dis*-ease. Ultimately, his doctor said it would have taken an [exercise stress test] to find the arterial blockage, ahead of time, (treadmill stress test and EKG).

Alberto's work ethic and workouts were legendary, going way beyond unconventional training to prepare his physiology for the stresses of competition, (some couldn't believe the intensity with which he trained and few others have ever trained in such grueling manners), but in hindsight, **Salazar said the component he neglected, even at his level of athletic development was the nutrition parts.**

You can push the body which makes it 'tougher' but to exercise doesn't keep the arteries cleaned out, especially with a genetic predisposition. In order to balance body chemistry, nutrition must be applied to get enough nutrition-density.

Reason 70. Yoga, Pilates & core training:

Even though these forms of resistance training are thought of as healthy, less stressful forms of exercise, they do increase the need for the B.N.B.B.s.

Remember, exercise is the stimulus for the nervous and hormone systems, but in order for them to carry out the signals, a surplus of nutrition-density (B.N.B.B.s) must be on board.

Every client I ever trained whom had been doing yoga, Pilates and core training were disappointed with the results they got from these exercise models, in terms of fat-loss and overall improvements to their physiques. Even though these exercise models are considered low-impact, the body still requires the B.N.B.B.s to support itself. These forms of exercise can be healthy, but they do not provide nutrition-density, to the body by doing them...you have to put the B.N.B.B.s in your body and then you'll get better results and feel better from these exercise forms.

Reason 71. Being underweight:

Often, the reason people are overweight relates to three possible main reasons; 1) lack of nutrition-density, 2) lack of absorption of calories and 3) lack of stability in the blood sugar levels (insulin resistance). With swings in blood sugar it's very difficult to gain healthy lean mass and maintain it.

In my case, when I was at my lowest of 4% body fat, I later realized I had misunderstood the importance of fats, mainly the good fats, on top of not understanding that just because I was eating 'clean' and taking *some* supplements, absorbing the supplements makes all the difference in the world. I did things *in*correctly for about 24-years, until I hit on a combination that I share with my clients today, to help them consistently get as good results.

Reason 72. Radiation:

Exposure to radiation sets up particular nutrition-requirements to help offset the damage that radiation can do to the body. The B.N.B.B.s help provide the nutritional building blocks, which help prevent catabolic effects (breaking down), while the body is trying to maintain balance.

Reason 73. Inadequate/inconsistent Whole-foods:

For whatever reason, some people don't eat enough Whole-foods. The B.N.B.B.s provide what an absence of Whole-foods misses out on. Whole-foods are supposed to be the basis of a healthy regime, but sometimes people need to get the nutrition-density, into their body, while they are learning how to shop, buy and prepare Whole-foods. B.N.B.B.s don't make up for an absence of Whole-foods, yet I have found that as nutrition-density builds up, in the brain and body, people begin to crave healthier and healthier foods, assuming the B.N.B.B.s were of high enough quality to do so.

Reason 74. Calorie/nutrient restrictive diets/skipping meals:

For whatever reason, some people restrict what they eat, restrict calories and skip meals. The Catch-22 is that the more one restricts calories the less nutrition-density they get, since food is the carrier of nutrition-density...*makes sense, huh!* I can't make people eat as much as they should for their goals, but I can offer really quick solutions that can help make up for the nutrition-density that is missing from their regime, with the B.N.B.B.s. I've known people whom were so concerned, almost phobic, about contaminants in their food that they start withholding a greater and greater amount of food until they get so weak, they can't walk across the street. The B.N.B.B.s make up for lack of nutrition-density, in the body when taken every day.

Reason 75. Men and women have some different nutritional-requirements:

There are some really easy improvements that can be made to improve how you feel. Whether you want to burn fat, gain strength, gain lean mass or improve endurance I can make a program specifically designed for you and you'll get better results than you've gotten before. Although there are some similarities between men and women and what their bodies require, men and women have some specific, different requirements, too. Just ask me for help!

Reason 76. Nutrition Diet Warning:

What we don't eat can be killing us:

NBC News reported on March 7, 2017. Lester Holt reported about *"...a new warning about your diet and startling news from doctors about what is associated with 1/2 of all fatal heart attacks and strokes...**that diet cited in 1/2 of heart attacks and strokes...**"*

"Doctors say there's a Whole range of superfooods that can help prolong your life."

"Heart disease, stroke, Type II diabetes...all major killers...now a new study finds almost 1/2 those deaths are associated with a poor diet (1-in-2 deaths)...the good food we don't eat as much as the bad food we do..," what the authors called a nutrition-crisis (see where this has evolved to?)...says NBC's Ann Thompson.

Dr. Dariush Mozaffarian, Freidman School of Nutrition at Tufts University says, *"Poor diet has now **surpassed tobacco smoking** as the number one cause of death and disability in this country."*

The study looked at 10-foods and found there are 4-types we need to avoid and 6 we need to eat more of.

"Most of the salt we eat is hidden in our food products," says Alissa Rumsey a Registered Dietician..."*...specifically the deaths were realted to the usual suspects, specifically too much salt and processed meat,"*..says NBC's Ann Thompson. But also a lack of nuts, seeds and seafood like salmon and tuna, rich in Omega-3 Fats (the good fats). *"Those are the kinds of fats that can really combat any kind of inflammation in our body...so they help to bring down your risk of heart dis-ease, diabetes, they have a lot of nutrients...fruits and vegetables are high in Potassium to control blood pressure and unsalted nuts, any kind...cashews, walnuts, and almonds offer unsaturated fats to help cholestrol levels...the key with nuts is moderation and portion size...a good place to start is thinking about adding one of these things into your day and slowly over time adding more nd more of these in,"* says Rumsey.

Thompson said to, *"... limit red meat, bacon and soft drinks to once or twice-a-week and dig into the right foods to ward off the wrong kind of problems."*

Reason 77. Sick all the time?

Catch every bug that comes along?

These are clear signs that the immune system is struggling to keep up. Apply all three-parts of a complete nutrition program and you may expereince a 50%-reduction in the number, frequency and duration of colds, flu and bugs that come along. You'll feel better more often.

I gurantee satisfaction with the B.N.B.B. programs I put together.

Prioritize your B.N.B.B.s

The order or priority of the nutrients, used by each person's body, may have variation, but everyone's body is made of the same basic nutritional building blocks. *Put the B.N.B.B.s in your body and let nature take over.* Not all supplements are created equal nor safe to consume. To learn what kind my decades of experience have steered me toward, contact me at the email in the appendix, for your complimentary consultation.

Fill out the pre-training questionnaire and email it to me to receive your free, hour consultation with me.

*"An exceptional trainer
teaches you how to think like them,
so you know what they know,..
so, you have them with you, for the rest of your life."*

Sovereign Valentine, June 2019

Pre-Nutrition Training Questionnaire:

Have you had professional, nutrition training before?__Yes___No

Are you coachable and open to Whole-foods nutrition suggestions?
___Yes ___No
Would you follow through on my suggestions?   ___Yes ___No

Did you know that your fitness/atheltic success or lack thereof is about 80%, based on the how well you apply the three parts of nutrition, during/from the first month, of your program?
___Yes ___No
Have you had professional B.N.B.B.s training?
___Yes___No

Are you coachable and open to suggestions about which B.N.B.B.s to take, for optimal results? (versus picking a program apart).
___Yes ___No

Currently participating in a structured, resistance-training?
___Yes___No
If so, frequency/duration of
sessions?____.
Have you had professional personal training before? ___Yes___No

Have you had fat-burning cardio-respiratory training before?
___Yes___No

Is it realistic for you to prioritize 3-4 hours [each week] to exercise?   ___Yes___No

What is your current bodyfat percentage?_______________________.

How much fat do you want to lose?_______________________.

What have been your biggest challenge(s)?

____.

Pre-Nutrition Training Questionnaire continued:

Are you committed to applying yourself to resistance-training, cardiovascular-training, and the 3 parts of nutrition: (1) Whole-foods, 2) Functional-foods, & 3) The B.N.B.B.s *for at least one year?* (versus a person whom starts stuff, but doesn't follow through).   __Yes ___No

With a standard of 12-20 pounds per month, how long could it take you to lose amount of fat, you intend to lose?________________________.

How many different weight-loss programs have you tried, before?

____.

I look for people whom have tried a few things that didn't work and whom are looking for something that definitely works. Are you the type of person whom wants a structured program that tells you exactly what to do throughout the day, so nothing is left to chance?

                                        ___Yes ___No

Are you willing to get your B.N.B.B.s squared away, from the beginning of your program?

                                        ___Yes ___No

Although you will likely begin to see and feel positive improvements right away, permanent fat-loss requires a lifestyle change. Are you willing to become more fit by committing to a program that definitely works, for at least one year? (Versus a short-term quick fix).

                                        ___Yes ___No

How long have you been wanting to lose weight?

____.

Imagine you have lost all the fat you ever wanted to, have more energy and look better than ever and all that is taken care of. In what way(s) would your life improve, as a result?

____.

*You may find it helpful to remove these pages, scan them and email them to me to assist with your complimentary consultation.

Afterword

How I like to work is to do an initial consultation/interview, with people whom want my help. During this time, I screen people for particular-characteristics, which indicate if this is a good program match for them or not, explain my fees, what is expected and so forth. I accept clients whom agree and commit to applying the nutrition-principles I teach, for at least one-year. If you don't want to make a one-year commitment I don't want to waste your time…this is not a quick-fix program, but rather a long-term, health-building program. I am a fairly tough trainer, since clients expect a lot for their money and in-turn, I expect accountability, so you get your money's worth...but, these are some of the reasons my clients get such good results. I only expect clients to do and apply what I personally apply myself.

How I know a person is serious and ready to be a client and how I take you seriously is when you get your Whole-foods, Functional-foods and B.N.B.B.s lined up, for at least weeks in advance. You have to have your supplies ready in advance and replenish them before you run out. This is sometimes considered a serious program, since there's no days that go by that you aren't sticking to the plan. You're either in/on it or you're not.

This program is considered Choice/Program #3 in my book *If I Were Her Trainer*, Amazon (2016). For people whom want increased strength, cardiovascular-fitness and conditioning, combining this program with a custom-designed resistance training program & fat-burning cardiovascular training is considered Choice/Program #4 in my book *If I Were Her Trainer*.

Once I'm convinced you're serious and a good candidate, and you've purchased a copy of this book you'll can receive a shopping list, along with a proposed program, to help make sure you have everything you need to succeed and get the most from each of your eight-week cycles.

Contact me via email and we'll set up a preliminary phone appointment from there. If you choose to hire me as your trainer to get going on this program, I'll be in consistent contact with you, to make sure you're on track and answer your questions, offer morale support and help you succeed on your program.

One of the most commonly asked question by my clients, after a few-weeks on this program is, "*Why are my hair, skin and nails looking so much better than they ever have before?*"

I look forward to working with you.

As a licensed health care provider, author, speaker and fitness professional I know from my own experiences what it feels like to want to improve my health, do what I think is right and still not get the kind of results I expected. I am sure you have your own goals and are looking forward to achieving them. I believe you are capable of living the life of your dreams in your healthy, ideal-self body and you will achieve your dreams.

I want you to contact me today and tell me about all the positive benefits you have experienced, as a result of this information!

In my experience, the greatest potential problem is in not educating yourself about it, but in simply doing it.

I cannot wait to hear from you. I especially cannot wait to share your success story with others.

-Sov

Appendix

Contact Information:

For a complimentary hour consultation, contact me at:

e-mail: sovereignmv@gmail.com

My blog:

https://sovereign-valentine.mykajabi.com/blog

Sovereign Valentine

CFT, CET, Yft, SSC, SPN, Cft, GFI, SFI, EMR, CERT, CMCht, Reiki Master

Reasons or Results! Training Systems ©2019

9 781717 178985